A self-help guide feeling better

Wendy Green

Foreword by Joanne Sale, senior lecturer in
mental health, University of Bedfordshire

PERSONAL HEALTH GUIDES

vie

ANXIETY: A SELF-HELP GUIDE TO FEELING BETTER

First published in 2010 as *50 Things You Can Do Today to Manage Anxiety*
Reprinted 2011, 2013
This revised edition copyright © Wendy Green, 2016

Vie Books is an imprint of Summersdale Publishers Ltd

Summersdale Publishers Ltd
46 West Street
Chichester
West Sussex
PO19 1RP
UK

www.summersdale.com

Printed and bound by CPI Group (UK) Ltd, Croydon, CR0 4YY

ISBN: 978-1-84953-822-0

Substantial discounts on bulk quantities of Summersdale books are available to corporations, professional associations and other organisations. For details contact Nicky Douglas by telephone: +44 (0) 1243 756902, fax: +44 (0) 1243 786300 or email: nicky@summersdale.com.

Disclaimer
Every effort has been made to ensure that the information in this book is accurate and current at the time of publication. The author and the publisher cannot accept responsibility for any misuse or misunderstanding of any information contained herein, or any loss, damage or injury, be it health, financial or otherwise, suffered by any individual or group acting upon or relying on information contained herein. None of the opinions or suggestions in this book are intended to replace medical opinion. If you have concerns about your health, please seek professional advice.

To my husband, Gordon, and my brother, Keith

Acknowledgements

I'd like to thank Joanne Sale, senior lecturer in mental health at the University of Bedfordshire, for kindly agreeing to write a foreword. Thanks also to Jennifer Barclay for commissioning this book and to Anna Martin, Sarah Scott and Sophie Martin for their very helpful editorial input.

Contents

Author's Note

We all feel anxious from time to time, for example, before sitting an important exam or giving a public speech. This may be partly because our lives are increasingly busy, with many people combining full-time jobs with raising a family and perhaps caring for elderly parents; there are also many other aspects of modern life that people find stressful. When we are feeling under pressure, it's natural to feel anxious. I am normally a fairly calm person, but I do become anxious sometimes – usually when I'm feeling as though I have too much to do. I've also noticed that I often worry about what might happen, rather than what is happening.

I've found that an effective way to banish anxiety is to focus on dealing with what is important now, rather than thinking about something that hasn't happened yet and perhaps never will. I also find that taking good care of myself by eating well and exercising helps me cope better when I'm feeling under pressure.

As with most conditions, there is no magical formula that will work for everyone with anxiety. However, I believe that an integrated approach, combining dietary and lifestyle changes – with modifications to the way you think and behave – and appropriate supplements and medication where necessary, offers the best chance of relief from anxiety for most people.

Wendy Green

Foreword

In its clinical guidelines on the management of anxiety, the National Institute for Health and Clinical Excellence (NICE) states that anxiety disorders are 'neither minor nor trivial'. It goes on to suggest that experiencing anxiety disorders can cause the sufferer great distress and that this can be persistent. Self-help – encouraging individuals to take responsibility for their well-being – is now being promoted as a way of overcoming anxiety, so any book that can help individuals who are prone to anxiety is to be welcomed. I believe that I would have found this a very useful resource, had it been available during the period of anxiety I experienced when my mother was dying.

This book offers people who are suffering from anxiety clear and current information and approaches. It manages to balance complementary approaches (where the evidence is often anecdotal) with the frequently predominant medical model (with its focus on evidence based on research findings). In doing this, it provides a comprehensive range of explanations and strategies, thus enabling the discerning reader to try out a multitude of options.

This book is written in a manner that allows the reader to dip in and out of it, while focusing on the particular approaches that may interest them. Its explanations are brief but precise, making it easy to follow, in particular during periods of anxiety or panic.

Many of the approaches discussed in this book may seem to be common sense, but these are often the things that we forget, and the benefits of being reminded of these is this book's strongest asset.

Joanne Sale,
senior lecturer in mental health, University of Bedfordshire

Introduction

According to a YouGov survey of 2,330 UK adults (aged 18 plus) commissioned by the Mental Health Foundation in 2014, almost one in five people feel anxious nearly all of the time, or a lot of the time. A further 41 per cent of people feel anxious some of the time. Women are more likely to be affected than men, with 22 per cent reporting feeling anxious a lot or all of the time compared to 15 per cent of men.

The survey found that the commonest causes of anxiety are:

- Financial issues – half of those who said they feel anxious in their everyday lives blamed money worries.

- Welfare of loved ones – was mainly a concern among women and older people.

- Work – four in ten employed people said they felt anxious about work issues.

- Unemployment – around one in three people not in work reported anxiety.

- Personal relationships – were mainly a source of anxiety among young people.

- Growing old and death – was a concern (unsurprisingly) among older people.

Age seems to be a major factor in anxiety; the Office for National Statistics reported in 2013 that people aged between 35 to 59 suffer the highest levels of anxiety, while the Mental Health Foundation's survey found that anxiety levels tend to fall with age, with almost half of 55-year-olds or over saying they rarely or never feel anxious. Despite the slight overlap in age groups reporting the most and least anxiety, these findings back those of other studies – in general, older people are the happiest and least anxious. This is probably down to the fact that they are less likely to have work and family responsibilities, and have fewer financial burdens.

The Mental Health Foundation's report of the findings, called *Living With Anxiety: Understanding the role and impact of anxiety in our lives,* reveals that many people said they feel more anxious than they used to and that society is more anxious than it was five years ago.

Another report published by the Mental Health Foundation in 2009, called *In the Face of Fear*, concluded that 'a culture of fear', fuelled by the media and public bodies over-exaggerating the threat of negative events, such as violent crime, terrorism, economic problems, disease and global warming, is at least partly to blame for the increasing levels of anxiety in the UK.

There is a strong link between anxiety and depression and physical health problems, such as asthma, allergies, a weakened immune system, gastrointestinal problems, migraines, arthritis, raised blood pressure and heart disease. There is also new evidence of a link between stress and Alzheimer's disease.

Experts believe that this is a result of the physical effects that stress has on the body. Also, people with anxiety often adopt unhealthy habits like smoking, drinking too much alcohol, and consuming too many sugary, refined foods and drinks containing caffeine to help them cope. Research suggests that a poor diet can be a contributing factor in unstable moods, anxiety and depression.

This book explains how social, biological, psychological, genetic and lifestyle factors can all play a part in anxiety. It offers practical advice and a holistic approach to help you manage your symptoms. You'll discover how eating a balanced diet rich in the nutrients needed for good mental health and taking regular exercise can help reduce anxiety. You'll learn strategies to help you manage stress and relax, as well as exercises to enable you to change unhelpful thoughts and behaviours. Information about appropriate supplements and medications, and techniques from complementary therapies that may be beneficial, are also included. At the end of the book, you'll find recipes based on the dietary guidelines, as well as details of helpful products, books and organisations.

Famous anxiety sufferers

- Ulrika Jonsson admitted that she had experienced depression and panic attacks (which are linked to anxiety) in the past. She says that she manages her condition with support from her family and friends, and by having a healthy, active lifestyle.

- Actress Patsy Palmer experienced a severe panic attack on her way to work one day, then woke up in a clinic the following morning with no recollection of getting there. At the time, she was trying to juggle the demands of single motherhood with a leading role in EastEnders. She says she still suffers from 'tiny anxiety attacks', but that she now knows how to handle them. She finds that talking to her husband and friends helps, and she has learned how to relax and take better care of herself.

- David Beckham suffers from ataxophobia, an anxiety-related disorder that leads to an obsessive need to keep things neat and tidy. He admitted to arranging drinks cans symmetrically in the fridge and even going as far as throwing one away if there was an odd number.

- Cameron Diaz has an obsessive compulsive disorder that manifests itself as a fear of catching germs and makes her wash her hands frequently and push open doors using her elbows, to avoid touching door handles.

- The actress Uma Thurman is claustrophobic, which meant that while filming a scene where she was buried alive in *Kill Bill: Volume II*, she didn't need to use her acting skills to appear frightened.

- The best-selling author Marian Keyes revealed that depression has dogged her for years. She added: 'I get afraid and then I don't want to leave the house.'

Chapter 1

About Anxiety

This chapter explains what anxiety is and gives a brief overview of the different types and their symptoms. It also discusses the possible causes of anxiety, including the social, psychological, genetic, biological, lifestyle and environmental factors that may be involved.

1 Learn about anxiety

Anxiety is a feeling of worry, apprehension or dread. It is a natural reaction to situations we find stressful and is part of the 'fight or flight' response that helps us deal with demanding events like sitting an important exam or giving a speech. Mild, short-term anxiety can help us feel more alert and focused, as it causes the body to release stress hormones to help it deal with the perceived threat, but long-term anxiety has detrimental effects on the mind and the body.

Anxiety and depression

Anxiety and depression are often interlinked – according to the Office for National Statistics, mixed anxiety and depression is the most common mental health problem in the UK, affecting nearly

9 per cent of the population (around four-and-a-half million people). This is because anxiety can be both a cause and a symptom of depression. It is often difficult for a GP to determine whether a person has depression with anxiety symptoms, or an anxiety disorder that is making them feel depressed.

If you suffer from symptoms like low mood, feelings of sadness and hopelessness, tearfulness, irritability, appetite changes (eating more or less), fatigue, changes in sleeping patterns (sleeping more or less), and a lack of interest in things you normally enjoy doing, it is likely that you are suffering from depression. Usually, if you focus on relieving your depression, your anxiety symptoms will ease too. Whether your anxiety is making you feel depressed, or vice versa, the advice in this book aims to promote good mental health, and so should help you both beat anxiety and boost your mood.

Seasonal affective disorder

Seasonal affective disorder (SAD) is a form of depression that occurs when the days get shorter and we are exposed to less sunlight. Around one in 50 people in the UK suffer from 'full-blown' SAD but, according to NHS Direct, as many as eight out of ten people suffer from a less severe form, which is commonly known as 'the winter blues'. The symptoms include anxiety, mood swings and a reduced ability to deal with stress. The severity of these symptoms will depend on which form of the condition you are suffering from.

A lack of sunlight is thought to lower levels of a brain chemical called serotonin, which has an important role in regulating mood. It also reduces levels of vitamin D in the body (it is produced in the skin on exposure to sunlight) which some experts believe may also be involved in SAD and winter blues. Exposure to bright light – usually in the form of a light box – for 30 minutes daily has been shown to relieve the symptoms of SAD in as little as two weeks. For milder symptoms, it may be helpful to make sure that you get outside as much as possible during daylight. A dawn simulator alarm clock that mimics a natural sunrise can also be helpful (see Useful Products).

Common forms of anxiety

Feeling anxious about stressful events is normal, but if you feel anxious most of the time for no particular reason or have irrational fears, and as a result are unable to function normally, you are likely to have an anxiety disorder. There are various types of anxiety disorder – the following is an overview of the most common types and their symptoms.

Generalised anxiety disorder (GAD)

GAD is diagnosed when a person suffers from excessive worry and anxiety for most of the time over a period of six months, along with at least three of the following symptoms (or just one for a child):

- Restlessness, or feeling 'keyed up' or 'on edge'
- Fatigue
- Difficulty in concentrating, or the mind going blank
- Irritability
- Muscular tension
- Problems falling asleep or staying asleep, or having restless sleep

Other signs of anxiety can include:

Physical symptoms

- Rapid, shallow breathing
- Pallor
- Sweating
- Trembling
- Feeling faint
- Headaches
- Dizziness
- Dry mouth
- Palpitations
- Loss of appetite
- Excessive thirst
- Excessive urination
- Stomach ache
- Nausea
- Diarrhoea
- Painful or missed periods
- Panic attacks
- Wanting to go to the toilet more often
- Tingling in the hands and feet

Psychological symptoms

- Impatience
- Being easily distracted
- Being oversensitive to criticism
- A sense of dread or panic
- Fearing you may lose control and/or go 'mad'
- Thinking that you might die
- Fearing you may have a heart attack/be sick/faint/or have a serious illness
- Thinking that people are looking at you and are aware of your anxiety
- Feeling as though things are speeding up, or slowing down
- Feeling detached from your environment and the people around you
- Wanting to escape from a situation
- Loss of libido

Panic attacks

Panic attacks are a common symptom of anxiety disorders. A panic attack is a rapid build-up of overwhelming fear and can include several of the following symptoms:

- A pounding, irregular heartbeat
- Chest pains

- Breathing difficulties

- Dizziness

- Feeling faint

- Nausea

- A choking feeling

- Sweating

- Trembling or shaking

- A sense of imminent danger and the need to escape

- Feelings of unreality and detachment

- Fear of losing control

- Fear of blacking out

- Fear that you are having a heart attack

- Fear of dying

Panic attacks can be triggered by a traumatic event, such as bereavement or divorce, or a stressful life change, such as having children or moving house. Hyperventilation is frequently a feature of panic attacks that is caused by breathing too quickly: this disturbs the oxygen and carbon dioxide balance in the body, leaving you with insufficient carbon dioxide and too much oxygen and causing many of the symptoms described in the previous list. Most panic attacks last for around 2 minutes, but they can sometimes go on for up to an hour. Many sufferers become anxious in between attacks, because they worry about when the next one is going to happen.

Three easy ways to overcome hyperventilation

Next time you start over-breathing, try one of these instant fixes:

1. Hold your breath for as long as you can without feeling uncomfortable – usually this is for about 10–15 seconds. Repeat a few times if you can. This helps you retain carbon dioxide.
2. Breathe in and out of a paper bag – this makes you reinhale the carbon dioxide you have exhaled.
3. Go for a brisk walk or jog while breathing in and out through your nose – this helps beat the tendency to over-breathe.

Phobias

A phobia is an irrational fear of a situation, animal or object that generally does not worry other people; for example, going to the dentist, snakes or heights. An individual with a phobia will go to great lengths to avoid the cause of their fear and this can have a disruptive effect on everyday life and relationships – depending on the type of phobia. This evasion can range from not being able to touch the object of fear to not even being able to look at an image of one. When a person with a phobia is confronted with the thing they fear, they are likely to experience extreme distress and anxiety that may take the form of a panic attack. A child with a phobia may cry or have a tantrum – adult phobics are usually aware that their fear is excessive and illogical, but child phobics may not be. When someone develops a phobia, it is sometimes possible to work out where it has stemmed from; for example, being bitten by a dog in childhood can lead to a fear of dogs in adulthood. Phobias are categorised into five main areas:

Agoraphobia is the fear of leaving an environment you consider safe – this could mean being unable to go out of the house, or even leave a room, or only being able to travel within a specific boundary. Some agoraphobics can travel more widely if they are accompanied by someone they trust.

Claustrophobia is the fear of enclosed spaces, such as lifts, buses, trains, cinemas, theatres, tunnels, revolving doors, public toilets, etc. While it is normal to fear being trapped when you are in a threatening situation, a person with claustrophobia will be afraid even when there is no obvious danger. Claustrophobia is usually characterised by two underlying fears: fear of restriction and fear of suffocation. The condition can be triggered by a traumatic event, such as being stuck in a lift, or it can be a learned behaviour, for example, from growing up with a family member who suffers from the condition. Around 10 per cent of the population is likely to experience claustrophobia at some time in their lives.

Social phobia is the fear of any situation that involves meeting other people, even in the course of everyday activities like going shopping, catching a bus, or walking into a room full of people. Sufferers feel excessively self-conscious and embarrassed; they may blush or sweat in the presence of others and feel tongue-tied. The condition can make holding down a job and having a social life very difficult and, if left untreated, sufferers can become more and more reclusive and isolated.

Blood or **injury phobia** is the fear of the sight of blood or injections, blood pressure measurement, or surgery. As a result, sufferers avoid visiting the doctor or dentist.

Simple phobia includes the fear of animals, birds, insects and specific objects, such as buttons, bridges, telephones, etc.

Other common phobias include a fear of vomiting, a fear of the dark, a fear of some part of the body looking or smelling wrong (an extreme form of social phobia), a fear of heights and a fear of fire.

One type of phobia can often lead to another, for example, someone with social phobia may develop agoraphobia because of their fear of meeting people, while someone with claustrophobia may develop a fear of flying and travelling by car, train or bus, because of their fear of enclosed spaces. Cognitive behavioural therapy (CBT) is an effective treatment for phobias (see chapter 6).

Proper terminology for the UK's most common phobias

- Arachnophobia (fear of spiders)
- Social phobia (fear of social and public situations)
- Aviophobia (fear of flying)
- Agoraphobia (fear of public or open spaces)
- Claustrophobia (fear of enclosed spaces)
- Emetophobia (fear of vomiting)
- Acrophobia (fear of heights)
- Carcinophobia (fear of cancer)
- Brontophobia (fear of thunderstorms)
- Necrophobia (fear of death – other people's or your own)

Obsessive compulsive disorder (OCD)

OCD is a condition characterised by obsessions or compulsions, and very often both. An obsession is a repetitive, involuntary, fearful thought about things like dirt and germs (contamination), harming oneself or others, throwing things away, or an abnormal concern with order and symmetry. Other common obsessions include abhorrent, blasphemous or sexual thoughts, or fears that things are unsafe. Most of us experience similar thoughts – for example, wanting to double-check you have switched off the iron or locked the front door – but these are normal reactions to everyday concerns about safety and security.

OCD sufferers are likely to experience such thoughts frequently in their daily lives yet, despite this, many are able to hide their condition and appear to function perfectly normally. At the other end of the scale, however, severe OCD can make it difficult to have normal relationships, hold down a job or socialise.

A compulsion is a repetitive physical action or mental ritual that temporarily reduces an obsession, for example, excessive cleaning and washing, checking, counting, hoarding and arranging objects. Compulsions can also involve repeating certain words or phrases, or praying. OCD sufferers don't act out their unpleasant thoughts and they are not a danger to others.

Around 1 to 2 per cent of the UK's population is thought to suffer from OCD and it seems to affect men and women equally. The condition tends to affect men in their late teens and women in their early 20s – but many people develop symptoms during childhood. Sufferers tend to go undiagnosed for many years, often because they are unaware they are suffering from a recognised condition, or from fear that they will be labelled as 'mad'.

Research suggests that OCD can run in families – this could be because of a genetic link or it could be down to copying the behaviour of an anxious parent. Other possible factors include a lack of the brain chemical serotonin, and negative thought patterns and behaviours. It is also thought that a traumatic event or excessive stress can trigger the condition in someone who already has a predisposition to it. Personality type may also be involved: perfectionists are thought to be more likely to develop OCD. Some research also suggests a possible link between a childhood bacterial throat infection, commonly known as 'strep throat', and OCD: it is thought that, in children with a genetic predisposition to the disorder, antibodies produced by the body's immune response affect the brain and trigger symptoms. Researchers believe that, when OCD is due to strep throat, it usually appears within one or two weeks of developing the infection.

Mild OCD often improves without treatment, perhaps when a stressful situation has been resolved. Cognitive behavioural therapy (CBT) has proved to be very successful in the treatment of moderate to severe OCD – although some sufferers may also need to take a suitable medication, such as an antidepressant called selective serotonin reuptake inhibitor (SSRI), which increases serotonin levels in the brain. For further details of these two treatments, see chapters 6 and 7. If you would prefer not to take medication, you may find supplements such as 5-hydroxytryptophan (5-HTP) or St John's wort helpful (see chapter 3).

Body dysmorphic disorder (BDD)

BDD is similar to OCD in that sufferers feel compelled to carry out particular rituals. With BDD, a person has a distorted self-image which leads to a preoccupation with what they perceive as defects in their appearance that go unnoticed by other people, such as bad skin or a big tummy; a sufferer won't go out in public without hiding their perceived defects first, perhaps with make-up or loose clothing.

Common rituals include frequently checking their appearance in a mirror, feeling their skin for blemishes, reapplying make-up and brushing their hair. Other compulsions can include constantly trying to improve one's appearance with new cosmetics and toiletries, exercising excessively and taking steroids. Around one in 100 people suffer from BDD and it seems to affect men and women equally. People usually develop BDD during their teens – although taking more interest in your appearance is considered part of growing up. In today's looks-obsessed society, it is considered normal to pay attention to one's appearance; however, when a person's concern with their appearance causes significant distress or handicap, it is likely they are suffering from BDD. The condition is often accompanied by social anxiety (because sufferers are worried about what other people will think about their appearance) and depression. BDD can sometimes lead to an eating disorder like anorexia, if a sufferer sees him or herself as being overweight. Like OCD, treatment for BDD usually involves CBT and sometimes SSRI antidepressants as well. This suggests that supplements that boost serotonin levels – such as 5-HTP and St John's wort – may also be helpful.

Post-traumatic stress disorder (PTSD)

PTSD is a mental condition caused by a traumatic event, such as a road, rail or air accident, or being the victim of a violent attack. A prime example is servicemen or women who have experienced combat – during world wars one and two the condition was known as 'shell shock'. Sufferers find themselves revisiting the event weeks, months, or even years later, through intrusive memories, flashbacks, hallucinations or nightmares.

The symptoms include intense anxiety and panic, depression, irritability, anger, an inability to concentrate, and sleep problems. In many cases, the symptoms ease within a few weeks or months. However, some people are affected for much longer and to the extent that they are unable to return to their normal lives. People in this situation will need professional treatment, which is likely to include CBT and taking SSRIs.

What causes anxiety?

There appears to be a number of factors involved in anxiety, rather than one specific cause.

Evolution

People experience anxiety because of evolution; although anxiety is an unpleasant experience, it has positive benefits that have been useful to humans throughout history. For example, when we are under threat or feel in danger (e.g. when you think you can hear a burglar), the body produces cortisol, adrenaline and noradrenaline, which make us feel more alert and anxious, and boost the heart rate to supply more blood to our muscles, to enable us to run away from or fight the burglar. So, from this perspective, anxiety is a natural and useful response in dangerous situations. Unfortunately, most of the anxiety we experience today is unlikely to be resolved by running away or fighting.

Society

Social factors, such as living alone and poverty, play a part in anxiety-related disorders. Research suggests that there are more people living alone than ever before – four times more than during the 1950s – as a result of higher divorce rates and fewer people choosing to marry. Single, divorced or separated people – especially lone parents – are more likely to suffer from anxiety disorders fuelled by loneliness and the pressures of surviving on a low income and bringing up children alone.

Gender

As we have already noted, more women suffer from anxiety than men. One reason for this is likely to be the hormonal fluctuations that occur during the menstrual cycle and during the menopause. Anxiety and panic attacks are common in women who suffer from premenstrual syndrome (PMS). PMS is the name given to a group of emotional and physical symptoms that some women experience during the days or weeks before their menstrual period.

Many women going through the menopause suffer from anxiety and depression as their ovaries dramatically reduce the amounts of oestrogen and progesterone they produce.

Keep a menstrual cycle diary

If you believe your symptoms may be due to PMS, note down what they are and when they happen for at least three months to see whether they could be linked to your menstrual cycle. If your anxiety symptoms are due to PMS or the menopause, the advice in this book is still likely to be helpful but, like anyone else, if your symptoms persist, you may want to seek medical advice.

Another reason for the higher incidence of anxiety-related disorders among women is that the social factors already mentioned are particularly likely to affect them. Lone parents are more likely to be female; more women than ever – both those who are part of a couple and those who are single – are juggling managing a home with bringing up children and working, which increases the likelihood of suffering from anxiety-related disorders. Many middle-aged women, labelled by the media as 'the sandwich generation', find themselves caring for ageing parents, as well as looking after their children, and going out to work. Women in this age group are more likely to experience loneliness following divorce, bereavement, childlessness, or their children leaving home.

Psychology

Psychologists believe that how we view ourselves and interpret events can help determine whether we suffer from anxiety or not. For example, a person with a negative view of themselves and the world is more likely to be anxious than someone with high self-esteem and a positive outlook. How much stress we experience and how we deal with it is also a factor; stress is thought to reduce levels of chemicals in the brain known as neurotransmitters, causing anxiety and low mood.

Genes

Research indicates that a tendency towards developing generalised anxiety disorder (GAD) and other anxiety-related disorders may be passed on genetically. In particular, genes linked to the way our bodies use the neurotransmitter serotonin have been implicated. However, when several family members behave in a similar way, it is possible that learned behaviours, such as copying the actions of a parent or other close family member, are involved. Shared lifestyles, for example the type of food a family eats and how active they are, may also play a part.

Abnormal brain function

According to Dr Daniel G. Amen, a leading neuroscientist and psychiatrist, and author of *Change Your Brain, Change Your Life,* anxiety is not just a psychological problem – it is also due to abnormal brain function. He says that how your brain works has a huge bearing on your mental health. According to Dr Amen, if the basal ganglia (large structures located deep inside the brain) are overactive, an individual is likely to be anxious and prone to panic attacks. He believes it is possible to calm down this part of the brain through positive thinking, relaxation techniques, cutting back on caffeine and alcohol, and using vitamin B supplements and aromatherapy.

Diet

Research suggests that a poor diet is linked to an increased risk of mental health problems, such as anxiety disorders and depression.

Other lifestyle factors

Using addictive substances, such as alcohol, caffeine and nicotine, can make anxiety worse, as can withdrawal from them.

Disconnection from nature

Some researchers believe that modern society's disconnection from nature is one cause of stress and mental health problems.

Life events

Some people develop anxiety after experiencing stressful life events – especially if they have a lot of pressures placed on them all at once. For example, if someone has work pressures, and financial and relationship problems all at the same time, it is hardly surprising if they become anxious. Anxiety is often due to feeling as though you can't cope with all of the demands placed upon you.

Also, people can learn to be anxious as a result of their past experiences. For example, if someone has previously suffered from bullying in the workplace, they are more likely to feel anxious when starting a new job.

2 Visit your GP

Anxiety can be a symptom of a number of physical conditions; for example, it can result from an overactive or underactive thyroid, ulcerative colitis and heart disease. Therefore, if you are suffering from anxiety, it is sensible to visit your GP to rule out any physical causes that may need medical treatment.

Anxiety can be short-lived, and by following the advice in this book and perhaps seeking specialist advice and support, you should hopefully be able to manage your condition. However, if your anxiety persists and affects the quality of your everyday life, your GP may refer you for counselling or psychotherapy, or prescribe a course of medication.

Don't suffer in silence

If your anxiety is accompanied by severe depression or suicidal thoughts or if you are contemplating self-harm, contact your GP or the Samaritans (see Directory), or go to your nearest A & E immediately.

Two anxiety sufferers' stories

Rachel, 25

Rachel was in her final year at university when the pressures of combining a full-time job with a degree course left her feeling stressed, depressed and anxious. She felt low, very tearful and was overwhelmed by the tasks she had to accomplish. In an attempt to make herself feel better, Rachel began taking St John's wort but stopped after a couple of weeks because she didn't feel any better, although she now recognises that she didn't give it a fair trial as she was 'looking for an instant cure'.

Her symptoms worsened and she explained that: 'Eventually I cracked and decided not to get out of the car to go into work. No matter how much I tried, I felt like my body was saying no.' She also recalled how, after angering another motorist while driving on a motorway, she returned home convinced that this person knew who she was and would come and find her so she hid beneath the bedcovers, crying. Realising she needed help, Rachel visited her GP. Her GP was sympathetic and agreed that Rachel's problems were due to the excessive pressure she was under. She was prescribed a mild antidepressant called Citalopram.

After speaking to her GP, family and friends, Rachel decided that she needed to make changes to her life to relieve the pressure she was feeling: 'I had to look at everything I was doing in my life and try to get a balance. My employer agreed to let me reduce my hours, which allowed me more time for studying and more time for me.'

She also used alternative therapies: 'Camomile essential oil was my best friend – I used to put it in oil burners and on hankies and it made me feel more relaxed. I also used Bach Rescue Remedy spray – when I felt anxious, I would spray it into my mouth and it helped.'

Rachel successfully completed her degree and was able to gradually stop taking the antidepressants. Since then she has found that exercise helps her cope with the stresses of daily life: 'I didn't try to exercise when I was going through my bad patch, as my life was so hectic. I now go to the gym regularly and, once I've been, I feel so much better.'

Keith, 54

Keith has experienced anxiety alongside bipolar disorder (a mental illness characterised by extreme mood swings) since the age of 17. He first became anxious when revising for his A-level exams, shortly before he was diagnosed with bipolar. Since then he has suffered from anxiety of varying degrees of severity during the depressive phase of his illness. His main symptoms are feeling worried and fearful. 'During the first few years after my diagnosis I used to suffer from panic attacks and was prescribed diazepam (a mild tranquilliser), which helped a lot. I don't take diazepam any more and fortunately don't suffer from panic attacks,' he explained.

'I tried deep-breathing exercises years ago, but decided I didn't need to do them because my medications helped me, but when I had problems sleeping, I used progressive relaxation – where you tense and relax your muscles – to relieve stress and help me drop off. I have also found walking helpful when I'm feeling anxious about something.'

What these two case studies illustrate is that anxiety can be treated in a variety of ways – it is simply a case of discovering what works for you.

Chapter 2

Eat an Anti-anxiety Diet

Most people are aware that there is a strong link between what we eat and our physical health, but the effect of our diet on our mental health seems to be considered far less.

Research by Mind and the Mental Health Foundation has shown that diet affects the brain's structure and the way it functions, and therefore influences mood and behaviour. The Mental Health Foundation's *Feeding Minds* report links the UK's rising levels of mental illness to our changed eating habits. For example, people eat around a third less fruit and vegetables, and less than half as much fish, than they did 60 years ago. These foods contain substances that the brain needs to function properly.

This chapter looks at how eating a balanced, low-glycaemic index (GI) diet can stabilise your blood sugar and help you deal with stress better, thus reducing anxiety. It also outlines the vitamins, minerals and fats you need for a healthy nervous system – including the antioxidant vitamins A, C and E; vitamin B complex; vitamin D; calcium; magnesium; selenium; iron; zinc; and essential fatty acids – and the foods that contain them. Protein foods and their role in the production of neurotransmitters (the brain's 'chemical messengers') are also discussed.

Some experts have linked anxiety and related conditions to caffeine, food and additive sensitivities; the main foods and additives thought to be implicated and the mechanisms involved are outlined in this chapter. There is also advice on how to determine whether food sensitivity is involved in your symptoms and what to do if you think it is. The importance of an adequate intake of water and how alcohol can affect mental health are also considered. You will find recipes incorporating many of these eating guidelines at the end of the book.

3 Choose low-GI foods

Your brain needs a steady supply of glucose (sugar) to enable it to function properly. Fluctuations in blood sugar levels can affect the brain, leading to moods swings, anxiety and even panic attacks. Also, when blood sugar levels are low, the body responds by releasing the stress hormone adrenaline, which not only stimulates the release of glucose, but also puts you on 'red alert', making you tense and anxious.

The glycaemic index (GI) is a measure of how quickly a food raises the level of sugar in the blood. Choosing foods with a low GI is thought to be the best way to maintain steady glucose levels and avoid emotional ups and downs.

Carbohydrates with a high GI are easily broken down into glucose, causing your blood sugar to rise rapidly and then fall just as quickly. Refined, processed foods, such as white bread, pastries, sugary drinks and sweets, tend to have a high GI. Carbohydrates with a low GI take longer to digest, so they cause your blood glucose to rise slowly and steadily. Unrefined, complex carbohydrates, like multigrain bread, porridge, wholewheat pasta, brown rice, sweet potatoes, carrots, beans, lentils, apples and bananas, have a low GI. It is thought that the fibre in these foods slows down glucose absorption.

Eating regularly also helps keep blood glucose levels stable. Munching on low-GI snacks in between meals, such as oat cakes and hummus, an apple, a banana, or a handful of nuts or seeds, can help prevent blood sugar peaks and troughs.

4 Eat more protein

Eating unrefined carbohydrates together with a little protein at each meal is especially beneficial to mental health: protein slows down the rate at which glucose is released into the bloodstream and unrefined carbohydrates help the brain absorb the tryptophan it contains. Tryptophan is an amino acid that the body uses to make serotonin, a type of brain chemical that is known as a neurotransmitter. Neurotransmitters transmit messages between nerve cells in the brain. Serotonin plays a part in the regulation of various processes in the body, including mood, and low levels of serotonin are associated with anxiety, depression and OCD. Good sources of tryptophan include turkey, chicken, fish, eggs, dairy foods, nuts, seeds, beans, lentils and wholegrains. Other foods containing tryptophan include bananas, avocados and dates.

A shortage of another neurotransmitter called gamma-aminobutyric acid (GABA) is also implicated in anxiety, as well as an inability to relax, irritability and self-criticism. GABA is produced in the body from glutamic acid found in various foods, including nuts, seeds, lentils, eggs, dark green vegetables – such as spinach – potatoes and bananas.

5 Increase your vitamin B intake

An adequate intake of B vitamins is essential for a healthy nervous system, as all B vitamins are involved in the control of tryptophan. Vitamin B1 (thiamine) deficiency is associated with low mood, irritability, generalised anxiety disorder (GAD) and phobias; vitamin B3 (niacin) is thought to relieve anxiety; insufficient vitamin B5 (pantothenic acid) has been linked to depression; vitamin B6 (pyridoxine) is needed by the body to produce both serotonin and GABA – a shortage can lead to nervousness, depression and irritability; and vitamin B9 (folic acid, or folate) deficiency is linked to anxiety and depressive symptoms. A study in 2009 suggested that middle-aged women with a low intake of folic acid and vitamin B12 were more likely to suffer from psychological problems: both are involved in the production of SAMe – a chemical the body uses to make neurotransmitters, such as serotonin. Insufficient biotin (a B vitamin which, confusingly, is sometimes referred to as vitamin H) has been linked with depression and panic attacks.

A balanced diet containing meat, fish, eggs, dairy foods, wholegrains, vegetables – especially green, leafy vegetables, beetroot and mushrooms – citrus fruits, pulses, nuts and seeds should supply enough B vitamins for most people's needs. If you're a vegan or you eat a lot of processed foods, you may be lacking in B vitamins, and if you're under stress, your body needs more of these nutrients: in such cases it may be beneficial to take a vitamin B complex supplement (see chapter 3).

6 Eat antioxidant-rich fruit and vegetables

Eating plenty of fresh fruit and vegetables will ensure that your diet is high in antioxidants, such as beta-carotene (a form of vitamin A) and vitamins C and E. Antioxidants are thought to neutralise the damaging effects that pollutants have on cells in the brain and the body. Fruit and vegetables also contain other nutrients, such as B vitamins and various minerals. Your body needs an adequate supply of these and vitamin C, in order to produce neurotransmitters. Eating a variety of different coloured fruits and vegetables helps ensure you obtain a wide range of nutrients and antioxidants. For example, the orange pigment in carrots, sweet potatoes and butternut squash supplies carotene; while another class of antioxidants called anthocyanin give fruits such as raspberries, strawberries, plums and blueberries their red, purple and blue colour.

7 Try mood-boosters from the kitchen cupboard

Did you know that some of the herbs, spices and fruits in your kitchen have relaxing or mood-boosting properties? Try some of these for a quick mental pick-me-up.

Basil-boost – this pungent Mediterranean herb is believed to both counteract anxiety and boost mood. Try adding torn basil leaves to pasta dishes and salads. Basil also brings out the flavour of summer fruits, such as strawberries, raspberries and blackcurrants – add a few finely chopped leaves to dishes like summer-fruit pudding, then garnish with a few whole leaves.

Chill out with chillies – eating chillies is thought to promote the release of relaxing endorphins. It might also help you fall asleep more easily during periods of anxiety, as chillies contain capsaicin, which research suggests may help regulate the sleep cycle. Use fresh chillies to spice up stir-fries and curries, as well as Mexican dishes, such as chilli con carne.

Tip

Wear disposable rubber gloves when chopping chillies, to avoid skin irritation. Avoid touching your eyes when handling them.

Lemon de-stresser – according to Japanese researchers, inhaling linalool – one of the substances that gives lemons their distinctive scent – dramatically reduces the body's stress response. So, next time you're feeling under pressure, try drinking freshly squeezed lemon juice in hot water. If you find the taste too sharp, sweeten with honey.

Relaxing rosemary – this aromatic herb is thought to improve mood and relieve mild depression and anxiety. Its distinctive taste goes well with meat, fish, vegetables and fruit, which makes it very versatile. Try adding rosemary sprigs to stews and casseroles; or spike meat, poultry or fish with rosemary, then brush with olive oil and bake in the oven. Alternatively, sprinkle sprigs of rosemary over new potatoes or mediterranean vegetables before roasting them in a little olive oil, or use a little finely chopped rosemary to enhance the flavour of fresh fruit salad.

Tranquil tarragon – tarragon is said to have calming sedative properties. Its delicate aniseed flavour goes well with fish and chicken. It also adds interest to salads and egg dishes – try adding a teaspoon of finely chopped tarragon to the egg mixture when making omelettes.

8 Get sufficient vitamin D

There is evidence that vitamin D deficiency can be involved in depression, and possibly seasonal affective disorder (SAD), because it is made in the skin after exposure to sunlight. This means you can become deficient in it during the winter, so it's important to obtain sufficient amounts from your diet.

A three-month trial at the Queen Charlotte's & Chelsea Hospital, in London, suggested that a diet rich in calcium and vitamin D reduced PMS symptoms, such as anxiety and depression, by about a third, as vitamin D helps the body to absorb calcium. Margarines, cereals and powdered milk are often fortified with vitamin D. Other good sources include oily fish, liver and eggs.

The recommended daily allowance is between 10 and 15 micrograms (400–600 international units). Vitamin D is only needed in very small amounts; therefore, it is usually measured in micrograms or international units. Be aware, however, that vitamin D is fat soluble, which means that any excess can be stored in the liver and fatty tissues. Overly high levels can be harmful and may even cause depression.

⑨ Mind your minerals

Minerals are essential nutrients that your body and your brain need in small amounts in order to function efficiently. Below is an overview of the minerals thought to be necessary for a healthy nervous system.

Calcium

Calcium deficiency has been linked to an inability to relax, nervous tension and irritability. The richest sources of calcium are dairy foods, in particular low-fat milk, hard cheese and yogurt. Tinned sardines are also a good source if you eat the bones. Good non-animal calcium providers include almonds; seeds; calcium-fortified soya products, such as tofu, milk and yogurt; seaweed; figs; dates; dried apricots; oats; Brazil nuts; watercress; leeks; parsnips; lentils; beans; and green leafy vegetables, such as kale and purple-sprouting broccoli.

To increase your absorption of the calcium they contain, sprinkle leafy green vegetables with a little ordinary vinegar. Drinking a tablespoon of cider vinegar and honey in warm water once or twice a day is also recommended for promoting calcium absorption.

'Good' bacteria – probiotics such as Lactobacillus – seem to improve calcium absorption. There are various probiotic foods and drinks available, such as Yakult and Activia.

Eating prebiotic foods, such as onions, tomatoes, leeks, garlic, cucumber, celery and bananas, which feed and encourage the growth of probiotics in the gut, could also help. Don't forget that calcium is also found in water – especially in hard tap water and some bottled waters.

It is recommended that your daily calcium intake doesn't exceed more than 2,000 to 2,500 micrograms. A higher intake may interfere with the absorption of other minerals, such as iron, and could lead to other problems.

Iron

A lack of iron is thought to contribute to low mood and anxiety. Women, vegetarians and dieters are most at risk of having low iron levels. Good sources include meat and green leafy vegetables.

Magnesium

Magnesium is a mineral often known as nature's tranquilliser. It is involved in the metabolism of B vitamins and essential fatty acids, and it helps the body absorb calcium. It also plays a part in the release of energy from foods and the transmission of nerve impulses. A lack of magnesium can lead to agitation and nervousness. Your magnesium levels may be low if you are stressed or eat a lot of sugary foods. Drinking a lot of coffee, tea or alcohol can also cause a deficiency, as this can have a diuretic effect, which increases the amount of magnesium excreted in the urine.

To ensure an adequate intake of magnesium in your diet, eat plenty of dark green leafy vegetables, such as spinach, broccoli and kale; seafood; tomato puree; nuts; seeds; wholegrains; beans, including baked beans; peas; potatoes; oats; and yeast extract. Another reason to avoid drinking too much alcohol (more than 14 units a week for women and 21 units for men) is that it can affect magnesium absorption. Fizzy drinks are also best avoided because the phosphates they contain also interfere with magnesium absorption.

Selenium

Research published in The Lancet in 2000 noted that a lack of the trace mineral selenium is associated with anxiety, depression and irritability. Selenium is thought to affect the way that neurotransmitters function, and is also believed to have antioxidant properties. Selenium-rich foods include wholegrains, Brazil nuts, cashew nuts, wheatgerm, eggs, fish, meat, poultry, garlic, mushrooms and brewer's yeast.

Zinc

A shortage of zinc in the diet has been linked with depression. Good sources of zinc include nuts, seeds, eggs, seafood, beans, and certain vegetables and fruit, such as mushrooms, broccoli, kiwis and blackberries.

10 Eat healthy fats

Your brain is around 60 per cent fat, so you need to eat sufficient fat for it to function efficiently; research suggests that diets that drastically reduce all types of fat in the diet can cause anxiety and depression. It's important that you consume the correct types of fat in the right proportions.

The foods we eat contain four types of fat – saturated, polyunsaturated (omega-3 and omega-6), trans, and monounsaturated (omega-9). Saturated fats are mainly obtained from animal sources, such as red meat, butter and full-fat dairy products. Polyunsaturated fats, also known as essential fatty acids (EFAs), are found in fish, vegetable oils, nuts and seeds. Trans fats are found in some margarines and processed foods, such as biscuits, pies and cakes. Monounsaturated fats are found in olive oil, rapeseed oil, avocados, nuts and seeds.

- Saturated fats are solid at room temperature and until recently people were advised to avoid them. However, research suggests that some of the saturated fats found in full-fat dairy products, such as whole milk, butter and yogurt, may boost health; they are thought to cut the risk of diabetes and heart disease and help weight management by keeping you full for longer. Butter (especially grass-fed) is also a good source of vitamin A.

- On the other hand, processed meats – especially sausages, bacon and burgers – should be eaten sparingly because they contain saturated fats that are linked with coronary heart disease and stroke, atherosclerosis (hardening of the arteries) and breast cancer. These types of saturated fats are also believed to make our brain cells less flexible and make it harder for the brain to use polyunsaturated fats.

- Polyunsaturated fats play a vital role in healthy brain function.

- Trans fats are also known as partially hydrogenated fats, because they are formed when vegetable oils are turned into solid fats, through a process known as hydrogenation. If you have a low intake of polyunsaturated fats and a high intake of trans fats, trans fats may replace polyunsaturated fats in the brain and this can have detrimental effects. They're also linked with hardened arteries, heart disease, diabetes and cancer, so are best avoided.

- Monounsaturated fats lower LDL (low-density lipoprotein) cholesterol and also have a role in brain function.

Polyunsaturated essential fatty acids (EFAs)

The fats and oils we eat are broken down into fatty acids. Some fatty acids can be produced by the body from other substances, but polyunsaturated fatty acids have to be obtained from food, hence they are known as essential fatty acids (EFAs). There are two main types of EFAs: omega-3, which is found in oily fish, nuts, seeds and some plant seed oils, such as flax oil and rapeseed oil, and omega-6, which is found mainly in plant seed oils, such as sunflower and rapeseed oil, corn oil and meat. Both omega-3 and omega-6 fatty acids are needed for the brain to function properly.

Long-chain and short-chain omega-3 fatty acids

There are two forms of omega-3 fatty acids: long-chain and short-chain. Long-chain fatty acids include eicosapentaenoic acid (EPA) and docosahexaenoic acid (DHA), which are found in oily fish, such as sardines, pilchards, mackerel, herring, salmon and fresh (not tinned) tuna. Research links the UK's lower intake of fish in recent years with a higher incidence of depression, including SAD, postnatal depression and bipolar disorder. Short-chain fatty acids, such as alpha-linoleic acid (ALA) are found in flaxseed oil, rapeseed oil, pumpkin seeds, sunflower seeds, almonds, walnuts, wholegrains, wheatgerm and soya beans. The body can also obtain EPA and DHA from these – although in smaller amounts.

Getting the balance right

Achieving the right balance between the two essential fatty acids is important, as too much omega-6 can interfere with the body's ability to break down omega-3 oils and has been linked with depression. British people's diets tend to contain too much omega-6, with a ratio of omega-3 to omega-6 of around 1:10 instead of 1:3, because many processed foods, cooking oils and margarines contain corn oil and sunflower oil. Therefore, you should aim to increase your intake of foods containing omega-3 oils and to cut down on products containing omega-6 oils, such as sunflower cooking oil and margarine, and use olive oil and olive oil-based margarines instead.

11 Drink plenty of water

Your brain needs sufficient water to function properly – even mild dehydration can affect mental well-being; symptoms of dehydration include restlessness and irritability. Experts recommend 1.5 to 2.5 litres of water daily, which can seem a lot, but remember that fruit and vegetables contain a lot of water and can contribute to your daily intake. Also, tea and coffee can be counted as part of your fluid intake; however, they contain caffeine, so it's advisable not to drink too much, or to choose decaffeinated versions instead.

12 Limit your alcohol intake

If you are stressed, anxious or depressed, it may be tempting to drown your sorrows with alcohol, because it can initially make you feel calmer; a recent UK survey suggested that people suffering from anxiety or depression were twice as likely to drink heavily. However, if you suffer from anxiety-related disorders, including depression, you should consider limiting your alcohol intake. This is partly because alcohol affects anxiety-reducing neurotransmitters such as GABA, but also because, when the effects of the alcohol wear off, you may be left feeling more anxious. Alcohol is a depressant, so it can exacerbate low mood, and its diuretic properties can disrupt your sleep patterns. It's also a toxin that your liver has to deal with using thiamine, zinc and other nutrients, leaving your reserves depleted. This is especially detrimental if you have a poor diet and already have low levels of these nutrients. Deficiencies in thiamine and other vitamins are often found in heavy drinkers and are linked to low mood, irritability and other psychological problems.

> **Drink responsibly**
>
> The recommended weekly alcohol intake is 14 units for a woman and 21 units for a man. One unit is roughly the equivalent of one small (125 ml) glass of wine, half a pint of beer or lager, one small glass of sherry or port and one single measure of spirits. For more information, visit www.drinkaware.co.uk.

13 Cut the caffeine

Caffeine boosts mood, improves alertness and concentration, and appears to cut the risk of dementia. However, too much has been linked to increased levels of the stress hormone adrenalin, anxiety and 'jitteriness'. So, if you consume a lot of caffeine-containing drinks and foods, such as coffee, strong tea, cola and chocolate, it may be worth reducing your intake. The caffeine content of tea and coffee can vary quite widely and depends on factors such as the brand, how much coffee/tea is used and how long it is left to brew.

Caffeine content of drinks/foods

Drink/food	Caffeine content (approx.)
Tea (mug)	55 mg–140 mg
Instant coffee (cup)	54 mg
Ground coffee (cup)	105 mg

Cocoa (cup)	5 mg
50 g plain chocolate	Up to 50 mg
50 g milk chocolate	25 mg

It is difficult to say how much caffeine is too much, as sensitivity to it varies from one individual to another; however, most experts suggest a daily limit of 300 mg.

Good substitutes for regular tea and coffee include herbal teas, redbush tea and decaffeinated coffee. Always wean yourself off caffeine gradually, to prevent withdrawal symptoms, such as increased anxiety and headaches. In the BBC series *The Truth About Food*, DJ David Sheppard, who confessed to relying on coffee to help him cope with his demanding early-morning starts, took part in a trial to see if drinking coffee benefited his mental performance. Without his knowledge, David was given decaffeinated coffee to drink for a week. Although David found that, initially, he was less alert, had a slower reaction time and his hands were less steady, by the end of the week he was functioning normally and found he felt less anxious, was sleeping better and had lower blood pressure.

14 Keep a food diary

For many people, eating a balanced diet, following a healthy lifestyle and dealing with stressful situations before they become a major problem will lead to an improvement in their anxiety symptoms. However, if your anxiety still persists, then it may be worth keeping a food diary to determine whether there is a link between what you eat and your symptoms. An ordinary notebook will do – simply note down every food you eat and any symptoms, such as increased anxiety, panic attacks, mood swings, problems sleeping, etc. Do this every day for four to six weeks and see if a pattern emerges. If your findings suggest that your anxiety symptoms are linked to food sensitivity, your next step should be to visit your GP.

15 Be aware of food sensitivities

Food sensitivity is complex but, in simple terms, there are two main forms: immediate and delayed. Immediate sensitivity is a true allergy, as it involves the immune response. Delayed sensitivity isn't a true allergy as it doesn't involve the immune response and is more likely to be caused by intolerance, otherwise known as non-allergic hypersensitivity.

A report in 2007 by Allergy UK claimed that around 2 per cent of the UK's population suffers from a food allergy and up to 45 per cent has some food intolerance, with one in ten of these people suffering from lethargy and anxiety as a result. Foods that have been linked with anxiety, depression and other psychological symptoms include wheat, dairy products, eggs, beef, sugar and caffeine. However, these views are controversial; in 2010, researchers at Portsmouth University argued that only one in ten people in the UK who believe they have a food allergy or intolerance actually have one. They warned that self-misdiagnosis could mean that people cut out certain foods unnecessarily and therefore risk nutritional deficiencies, and urged anyone who believed they had food-related symptoms to visit their GP.

Immediate sensitivity

Immediate sensitivity to food causes symptoms within an hour or two of eating the offending food. Where the reaction is severe, it's known as anaphylaxis. Here, the symptoms are much more pronounced – there may be swelling of the lips, mouth and tongue. In extreme cases, there may be a sudden drop in blood pressure and loss of consciousness – anaphylactic shock – that in extreme cases can lead to death. Some researchers believe that people who react in this way to certain foods may have a leaky gut wall that has become overpermeable, perhaps as a result of stress or irritants, such as coffee, alcohol or some medications. In this state, the gut wall allows partially digested molecules of food to enter the bloodstream, where they trigger a response from the immune system. Always seek professional medical help immediately if you suspect an anaphylactic reaction.

Delayed sensitivity

In delayed sensitivity, symptoms appear within 6 to 48 hours of eating the trigger food. This could be a result of low levels of certain digestive enzymes, such as lactase, which breaks down milk sugars (lactose). Another cause could be raised sensitivity to natural substances found in foods, such as salicylates (chemicals found mainly in fruit, herbs and spices), caffeine and histamine, found in foods such as strawberries, cheese and chocolate. Another possible cause is food additives – especially the artificial colouring tartrazine, the sweetener aspartame and the food flavouring monosodium glutamate. Some people may suffer from both immediate and delayed food sensitivity.

Testing for food allergies

There are two allergy tests your GP may perform to check for food sensitivities:

Skin-prick test

This test is useful for diagnosing immediate food sensitivity. A few drops of an extract of the suspected food(s) are applied to the skin – usually the forearm – then a small prick or scratch is made. If the area reacts by becoming red and itchy, it confirms sensitivity. Some experts claim that the test is unreliable because of difficulties in interpreting the results. However, a positive result suggests that food sensitivity is a possibility.

Note Where there has been an anaphylactic reaction to a specific allergen, skin testing may not be appropriate or necessary.

RAST test

Another test that is used to detect food sensitivity is RAST (radioallergosorbent test) otherwise known as the IgE antibody test. This measures the level of antibodies in the blood following intake of the suspected food. As this test measures IgE levels, it's an indicator of immediate food sensitivity – a true allergic reaction involving the immune system. It doesn't reveal delayed food sensitivity because it doesn't involve the production of antibodies. If a high level of antibodies is detected, it suggests that the ingested food could be causing a reaction. However, this test has been known to give the wrong results, and can only test for the common allergens, such as peanuts and eggs.

If the results of either test point to a food sensitivity, your GP may refer you to a dietician who may suggest following an 'exclusion and challenge test'.

Exclusion and challenge test

An exclusion and challenge test involves stopping eating the suspect food for two to six weeks to see if your anxiety symptoms improve. You'll then be asked to reintroduce the food (the challenge part) to see if your anxiety worsens again. Finally, you'll be asked to exclude the suspected foods to see if your anxiety lessens. Always carry out this process under the supervision of your GP and a dietician to make sure that you follow a balanced diet throughout the test period.

Online food directory for allergy sufferers

Select Food is an online directory of companies that sell foods for people with allergies, such as wheat-free and dairy-free products. For further details, see Directory.

16 Consider nutritional therapists' advice

Nutrition consultant and author Ian Marber, one of the founders of The Food Doctor, stresses the importance of maintaining steady blood sugar levels by avoiding sugary products and eating wholegrain foods. He recommends eating plenty of fruit and vegetables – especially tomatoes, lettuce, beetroot and beans – to ensure an adequate intake of B vitamins and the mineral chromium, which he says also help stabilise the blood sugar. He adds that cutting down on alcohol helps keep your blood sugar under control. He also emphasises the importance of omega-3 oils in the prevention of anxiety and depression, pointing out that tinned sardines and mackerel are much cheaper than fresh oily fish, but are just as rich in essential fats. Marber claims that a diet containing very high levels of protein has been shown to interfere with the body's production of mood-enhancing serotonin and suggests replacing meat with vegetable proteins – such as beans – tofu or yogurt.

Nutritional therapist Patrick Holford warns that our reliance on stimulants, such as caffeine, alcohol and nicotine, may give us an energy boost, relieve anxiety or help us keep going after a hard day's work, but the highs they provide can quickly disappear, leaving us prone to mood swings, anxiety and exhaustion. He argues that the best way to maintain a balanced mood is to reduce your intake of stimulants and to eat a healthy, balanced diet.

The anti-anxiety diet

In a nutshell, this is a balanced, wholesome diet containing wholegrains, oily fish, poultry, meat, low-fat dairy products, fresh fruit and vegetables, legumes (beans, peas and lentils), nuts, seeds, olive oil and plenty of water. These supply all of the key nutrients required for healthy brain function.

Chapter 3

Helpful Herbs and Calming Supplements

It appears that supplements are growing in popularity – in 2015, market researchers Mintel claimed that two in five adults in the UK take vitamins daily. They suggested that young adults turn to supplements because of the stresses of modern life, while older people take them because they are worried about the effects of ageing.

This chapter looks at the various herbal, vitamin and mineral supplements commonly recommended for the relief of anxiety and related conditions. For each supplement, there is information on its beneficial effects, how it works and evidence of its effectiveness, as well as advice regarding its safe use; it is important to remember that just because something is termed 'natural' it is not necessarily harmless. For example, the herbal remedy kava was traditionally used to relieve anxiety, until it was banned in the UK in 2003, amid reports of liver damage.

Do supplements work?

Supplements are often controversial, with some recent reports claiming that isolated substances don't provide the same benefits that nutrients found in foods do. However, for many of us, supplements represent a convenient means of improving our diets or increasing our intake of beneficial herbs, vitamins or minerals. Sometimes there is anecdotal evidence but no, or insufficient, conclusive evidence that a supplement works. This doesn't necessarily mean that it's ineffective – often it's just that the research hasn't been done. Even though the turnover in the herbal medicine sector is quite high, many individual manufacturers are unable to meet the high financial costs of clinical trials.

Sometimes the type of research undertaken gives results that are deemed inconclusive. For example, if a study is carried out on only one group of participants, without a comparison group to take a different treatment or not have any treatment at all, the results may be unreliable. Or, the participant might feel an improvement because they expect to, rather than because of the treatment itself, which is known as the placebo effect.

Randomised controlled trials (RCTs) are viewed as the most reliable type of trial because they randomly place participants in a treatment group or a control group. The treatment group receives the treatment under scrutiny, while the control group may receive a placebo or another treatment, for comparison. RCTs can be single-blind, where the participant doesn't know which treatment they are receiving, or double-blind, where neither the participants nor the researchers know who is receiving which treatment.

Another problem is that some herbal remedies have several active ingredients, and this can make it difficult to pinpoint which ones have the beneficial effects. Also, the quality of herbal medicines can vary quite a lot due to differences in plant species, the type of soil where they are grown, and methods of extraction and storage, etc. These differences can make it difficult to make any firm conclusions regarding particular herbs.

How safe are supplements?

Herbal products are usually sold in the UK as either traditional herbal registration (THR) remedies or herbal food supplements. THR products are regulated and monitored by the government agency known as the Medicines and Healthcare products Regulatory Authority (MHRA). If a product has a THR stamp it means the MHRA is satisfied it meets quality standards, has appropriate labelling and a product information leaflet. It also indicates that the herb has been used in traditional remedies for over 30 years. All THR products have a nine-digit registration number starting with the letters THR on the container or packaging.

Herbal food supplements come under the remit of the Food Standards Agency (FSA) and the Chartered Trading Standards Institute at local authority level, and are not under the same legal and manufacturing scrutiny. This means there is no guarantee of their content or quality. In 2015 the School of Pharmacy at University College London tested over 70 of the herbal remedies most often bought from the high street or online and found that while most contained high amounts of the main ingredient, worryingly up to a third had very little or none at all. So it is probably best to choose THR remedies or, if a product isn't registered, check that it is from a reputable company.

Also, a few herbal medicines have a product licence. Licensed herbal medicines, like any other medicines, are required to demonstrate safety, quality and effectiveness, and to provide guidelines on safe use. Only herbal medicines with medicinal claims supported by acceptable clinical data are given product licences. They can be identified by a nine-digit number, prefixed by the letters PL.

There is a full list of herbal medicines that have been granted a traditional herbal registration on the MHRA website, as well as further advice and information about using herbal medicines safely. The contact details are in the directory at the end of this book.

Safety issues regarding traditional Chinese herbal medicines

Traditional Chinese herbal medicines are currently unregulated; this has led to concerns regarding the quality and safety of some products. As a result of these issues, it is advisable not to use Chinese herbal products, at least until some form of regulation is introduced.

Inform your GP

Always inform your GP if you are taking a herbal supplement, as some can reduce the effectiveness of conventional drugs, or cause side effects. This is especially important if you have to undergo surgery, as some herbal medicines could cause complications.

17 Benefit from herbs and supplements

Here is an overview of the herbs and other supplements for which there is some evidence of effectiveness in the relief of anxiety and depression, and which are deemed safe to take. They are available in various forms, including tablets and tinctures; some of the herbs mentioned can be grown in your own garden and made into herbal infusions, or can be bought in teabag form. Related products are listed in the Useful Products section at the end of the book.

Camomile

What it is: a daisy-like plant from the Asteraceae (Compositae) family. The flowers are the part of the plant that is used. German camomile produces the biggest flowers, so it is more popular than Roman camomile in herbal medicine.

Beneficial effects: it relieves anxiety and promotes sound sleep.

How it works: camomile flowers contain the amino acid glycine, which is a muscle and nerve relaxant. Another active ingredient is a flavonoid called apigenin, which may enhance the calming effects of the neurotransmitter gamma-aminobutyric acid (GABA).

Evidence of effectiveness: a small study in 1998 suggested that German camomile was helpful in relieving anxiety, but the evidence was deemed inconclusive.

Safety: camomile is generally safe, although you should avoid taking it if you have an allergy to the Asteraceae (Compositae) family of plants, which includes aster, chrysanthemum, mugwort, ragweed and ragwort.

Available as: camomile is widely available as a tea. You can also make your own: grow camomile in a sunny spot, in pots or in the garden. Pick the flowers while in full bloom and hang them upside down in small bunches in a well-ventilated warm room until they are crisp and completely dry. Store the dried flowers in an airtight jar. To make up a cup of camomile tea, pour boiling water over one tablespoon of the dried flowers, cover and leave to stand for 5 to 10 minutes. Strain, add honey to taste, and drink while hot. Camomile tea has a distinctive, apple-like flavour. If you dislike the taste, try adding two or three bags to a hot bath to enjoy the benefits without having to drink the tea. Camomile is also available as a tincture.

Easy infusion

Use a cafetière to make your herbal teas quickly and easily. Put the herbs in and add boiling water. Replace the cafetière lid. Leave to brew, then press down the plunger and pour.

Gamma-aminobutyric acid (GABA)

What it is: GABA is a neurotransmitter and amino acid.
Beneficial effects: it has a calming, soothing effect on the brain.
How it works: it is thought to lower stress hormones and boost serotonin levels.
Evidence of effectiveness: two small studies, conducted by a maker of GABA supplements in Japan, concluded that GABA has an anti-anxiety effect. In the first study, the researchers found that taking GABA had a relaxing effect on brain waves. In the second study, people with a fear of heights were asked to walk across a narrow pedestrian bridge after taking a GABA supplement or a placebo. The participants who took the GABA supplement had lower levels of anxiety, which was measured by checking stress hormone levels in their saliva. However further, larger studies are needed.
Safety: if you are pregnant or breastfeeding seek medical advice before taking.
Available as: capsules (e.g. Eurovital Gaba Plus).

Hawthorn, Californian poppy and magnesium

What it is: hawthorn is a common hedgerow plant; Californian poppy is a golden flowered garden plant; and magnesium is a mineral. These three ingredients have been combined to produce an anti-anxiety supplement.

Beneficial effects: it helps relieve mild to moderate anxiety and insomnia.

How it works: the exact mechanism isn't known, but hawthorn and Californian poppy are believed to have sedative, anti-anxiety properties. A lack of magnesium is linked to various psychological symptoms, including anxiety and irritability. Magnesium may also aid sleep, because it relaxes the muscles.

Evidence of effectiveness: one large French RCT (randomised controlled trial) of 264 GAD (generalised anxiety disorder) sufferers in 2004 found that those who took a hawthorn, Californian poppy and magnesium supplement, called Sympathyl, experienced a greater reduction in anxiety symptoms than those taking a placebo. In a review of the evidence for or against herbal remedies for depression and anxiety in 2007, Edzard Ernst, professor of complementary and alternative medicine at Exeter University, described this remedy as 'promising'.

Safety: fewer than one in ten people in the study who took the supplement experienced mild to moderate side effects such as stomach upsets.

Available as: Sympathyl is made in France and doesn't appear to be available in the UK or the US. However, there is a supplement called ESI Passiflora and Valerian Plus that you can buy in the UK that contains hawthorn, Californian poppy, passion flower and valerian. You can also buy magnesium supplements, such as Magnesium B.

Hop

What it is: a British climbing perennial plant. The flowers are the part of the plant that is used.

Beneficial effects: they act as a sedative, relieve stress and encourage sound sleep.

How it works: hops appear to have a sedative effect on the central nervous system, but the mechanism involved is unknown.

Evidence of effectiveness: dried hops have traditionally been used to treat anxiety, restlessness and insomnia. One study reported that valerian and hops combined promoted good-quality sleep. The German E Commission recommends hops for the relief of restlessness, anxiety and mood disorders.

Safety: no side effects have been reported, however, hops can increase the effects of sedatives, sleeping tablets and alcohol, and have a mild depressant action, so they are not recommended for people with depression.

Available as: they are available as a tincture (e.g. Dormeasan) and tablets (e.g. Stressless and Kalms).

The German E Commission

This is an expert committee in Germany that reviews herbal drugs and preparations from medicinal plants for their quality, safety and effectiveness.

5-hydroxytryptophan (5-HTP)

What it is: 5-HTP supplements are usually made from the seeds of the griffonia plant, which comes from West Africa.

Beneficial effects: it boosts mood and relieves anxiety, including OCD and panic attacks, and also aids sleep.

How it works: the body uses 5-HTP to produce the neuro-transmitter serotonin. A lack of serotonin has been linked to depression and anxiety.

Evidence of effectiveness: one RCT tested 5-HTP as a remedy for anxiety disorders: 45 participants suffering from agoraphobia with panic attacks, GAD, panic disorder or OCD were randomly given clomipramine (a tricyclic antidepressant), 5-HTP or a placebo for eight weeks. Those who took 5-HTP also received 150 mg of carbidopa (a drug that increases dopamine in the brain) per day. Five of the 15 people who took 5-HTP improved by more than 50 per cent, compared with only one out of the 15 taking the placebo. Another RCT involving 24 sufferers of panic disorder reported that those taking 200 mg of 5-HTP 1.5 hours before being subjected to a 35 per cent CO_2 challenge experienced fewer panic and anxiety symptoms than those taking a placebo. Several RCTs have suggested that 5-HTP supplementation helps people fall asleep quicker and stay asleep for longer.

Safety: 5-HTP should not be taken with SSRI antidepressants, such as Prozac, weight control drugs, or if you are pregnant. Some people may experience a temporary worsening of anxiety symptoms before noticing an improvement.

Available as: tablets (e.g. 5-HTP 100 mg, Serotone 5-HTP and Solgar 5-HTP).

What is a 35 per cent CO_2 challenge?

A 35 per cent CO_2 challenge involves participants inhaling one or two breaths of air, of which 35 per cent is carbon dioxide (CO_2). Studies have shown that people who suffer from panic attacks tend to be hypersensitive to carbon dioxide and they experience panic-like symptoms when they inhale it. A 35 per cent CO_2 challenge is sometimes used to induce panic attacks in sufferers taking part in research into the condition.

Lemon balm

What it is: a white-flowered plant with lemon-scented leaves that is part of the mint family. Also known as Melissa officinalis.

Beneficial effects: it helps reduce anxiety and irritability, as well as associated insomnia and headaches. This herb is approved for 'nervous sleeping disorders' by the German E Commission.

How it works: it is thought to stimulate the production of neurotransmitters and may offset the effects of caffeine.

Evidence of effectiveness: lemon balm has traditionally been used to ease nervous tension and anxiety, and to promote sleep. A study in 2004 suggested that it had short-term anti-anxiety effects on healthy volunteers.

Safety: may cause drowsiness – if affected, don't drive or operate machinery.

Available as: teabags (e.g. Salus House Lemon Balm Teabags) and a tincture (e.g. from G Baldwin & Co). You can also make your own tea: lemon balm can be grown in a sunny or part-shaded spot in a large pot or in the garden and needs well-drained soil. Pour boiling water over one tablespoon of fresh (or one teaspoon of dried) lemon balm leaves. Leave to brew for 5 to 10 minutes, then strain, sweeten to taste with honey, and drink while hot. If you don't like herbal teas, try adding finely chopped leaves to fish or meat dishes. They also taste great blended into a melon or pear smoothie.

Omega-3 essential fatty acids (EFAs)

What they are: EFAs are fats that the body needs for various functions but can't produce itself. Omega-3 EFAs are found in oily fish, nuts, seeds and seed oils; if you don't consume these foods regularly, a supplement may be beneficial.

Beneficial effects: omega-3 EFAs reduce symptoms of depression and may enhance the effects of antidepressants and ease anxiety.

How they work: omega-3 EFAs provide eicosapentaenoic acid (EPA) and docosahexaenoic acid (DHA), which brain cells need in order to function efficiently.

Evidence of effectiveness: many studies suggest that omega-3 EFA supplementation can reduce depression. In 2007, a review of RCTs examining the effectiveness of omega-3 EFA supplementation in treating mental illness concluded that there was good evidence that omega-3 EFAs reduced symptoms of depression and some evidence that they may also ease symptoms of anxiety.

Safety: omega-3 EFAs can interact with blood-thinning drugs such as warfarin. The recommended daily amount for mental well-being is 1,000 mg of EPA/DHA. Both fish oil and cod liver oil are good sources of EPA and DHA. Cod liver oil also contains vitamin D, which many people in the UK are deficient in (because the leading source is sunlight), and vitamin A. However, it is advisable not to take cod liver oil alongside a multivitamin, as any excess is stored in the liver; too much of these vitamins can be harmful. Alternatively, if you are a vegetarian, you could take flaxseed oil, but the body obtains less EPA/DHA from plant sources.

Available as: oil (e.g. Seven Seas Pure Cod Liver Oil Liquid) and capsules (e.g. Pulse Omega-3 Pure Fish Oils).

Passion flower

What it is: passion flower is a climbing shrub with purple and white flowers that is native to South America and popular with gardeners in the UK. Both the flowers and leaves can be used. It is also known as passiflora.

Beneficial effects: passion flower combats stress and supports the body during periods of anxiety. It is also a traditional South African remedy for insomnia – especially for people who have trouble staying asleep.

How it works: its active ingredients are alkaloids, which have mildly sedative effects, possibly by enhancing the effects of the neurotransmitter GABA.

Evidence of effectiveness: very little research has been done on the effectiveness of passion flower in treating anxiety, but one small double-blind RCT in 2001 found it to be as effective as the tranquilliser oxazepam in the treatment of GAD, but with fewer side effects.

Safety: passion flower may occasionally cause dizziness, confusion, heart problems and inflammation of blood vessels. Very rarely, there may be severe toxicity, even with normal doses. Do not take passion flower if you are pregnant or breastfeeding.

Available as: tablets (e.g. RelaxHerb), a liquid extract (ESI Passiflora and Valerian Plus) and a tincture (e.g. from G Baldwin & Co and Napiers).

Rhodiola rosea

What it is: Rhodiola rosea is an extract from the rhizome and root of the Rhodiola plant, which grows in Scandinavia, Canada, Siberia and northern China. It is also known as golden root or roseroot.

Beneficial effects: it relieves symptoms of stress, such as mild anxiety, and boosts concentration.

How it works: the active ingredients are rosavins, which increase tolerance of physical, mental and environmental stress by acting on the hypothalamus in the brain. They may also improve the transportation of tryptophan and 5-HTP to the brain.

Evidence of effectiveness: various animal, laboratory and human studies have shown that Rhodiola rosea can help increase stress tolerance. A pilot six-week-long study, published in the *Journal of Alternative and Complementary Medicine*, in 2008, suggested that a daily dose of 340 mg of Rhodiola rosea extract significantly reduced anxiety levels in ten participants who had been diagnosed with GAD.

Safety: do not take Rhodiola rosea if you are pregnant or suffer from kidney or liver problems.

Available as: tablets (e.g. Vitano), capsules and alcohol-free extract.

SAMe

What it is: S-adenosyl-methionine (SAMe) is a chemical compound found in the body. It is derived from methionine, an amino acid found in protein foods, and adenosine triphosphate (ATP), a substance involved in the production of energy in the body. It is also known as s-adenosylmethionine.

Beneficial effects: SAMe helps relieve depression.

How it works: it is used by the body to make neurotransmitters, such as serotonin.

Evidence of effectiveness: a report reviewing the evidence regarding the effectiveness of complementary and alternative therapies for depression, published in the *Journal of Affective Disorders* in 2006, concluded that SAMe might offer some benefit to people with depression. The report cited evidence from two previous reviews – one which pooled the results of seven RCTs and claimed that SAMe was as effective as tricyclic antidepressants (TCAs) – see chapter 7 – in the treatment of depression. However, the authors of the report cautioned that most of the RCTs lasted for less than six weeks and some used flawed research methods.

Safety: SAMe should not be taken by people with bipolar disorder, as it may cause mania. If you are taking antidepressants, strong painkillers, or blood-thinning medications, such as aspirin, heparin and warfarin, speak to your GP or pharmacist before using it.

Available as: tablet form (e.g. SAMe by Biovea).

Skullcap

What it is: skullcap is a violet-flowered plant native to the US. It is also known as hoodwort.

Beneficial effects: it relieves nervous tension and anxiety, and aids sleep. It was listed as a tranquilliser in the US Pharmacopeia in 1863.

How it works: research suggests that this herb may enhance the effects of the neurotransmitters GABA and serotonin.

Evidence of effectiveness: skullcap has traditionally been used as a natural tranquilliser and to relieve insomnia. A double-blind, placebo-controlled study, published in the American journal *Alternative Therapies in Health and Medicine* in 2003, suggested that skullcap has anti-anxiety properties.

Safety: skullcap is safe when no more than than 6 g is taken daily. Excessive consumption can lead to liver damage; anyone with liver damage should therefore avoid taking skullcap. Pregnant women should not take this herb, nor should anyone who is taking benzodiazepines or barbiturates.

Available as: an alcohol-free liquid (e.g. Skullcap, Oat and Passionflower Compound), a tincture, tablets (e.g. Stressless) and capsules (e.g. Nature's Way Skullcap Herb).

St John's wort

What it is: St John's wort is a hedgerow plant with yellow flowers.
Beneficial effects: it relieves moderate to mild depression and may also be helpful for anxiety and OCD.
How it works: the active ingredient hypericin is thought to keep the chemicals linked to positive mood, such as serotonin and norepinephrine, in the brain for longer by blocking the effects of an enzyme that destroys them.
Evidence of effectiveness: several studies lasting between one and three months report that St John's wort is more effective than a placebo and is as effective as tricyclic antidepressants (TCAs) in the treatment of mild to moderate depression. Some evidence suggests that St John's wort may also be just as effective as SSRI antidepressants in the treatment of mild to moderate depression, with the added benefit of fewer side effects. There is only anecdotal evidence that St John's wort eases anxiety and only weak evidence that it helps OCD.
Safety: if you are taking any kind of medication, seek advice from your GP or pharmacist before taking St John's wort, as it can react with several commonly prescribed drugs, including the contraceptive pill, antiepileptic drugs, warfarin and the antibiotic tetracycline. It can enhance the effects of SSRI antidepressants and should not be taken by anyone with bipolar disorder. It can also increase sensitivity to sunlight.
Available as: tablets (e.g. Kira St John's wort), capsules and a tincture.

Valerian

What it is: valerian is a plant with pink and white flowers that is sometimes known as 'nature's Valium'. The root is the part used in herbal medicine.

Beneficial effects: it may help relieve stress, anxiety, depression and insomnia.

How it works: valerian seems to promote the production of neurotransmitters such as GABA. It may also neutralise the effects of caffeine.

Evidence of effectiveness: valerian is a traditional herbal remedy for anxiety. It is approved by the German E Commission for use as a mild sedative. Some studies have suggested that valerian may relieve anxiety and others have not. In 2006, a systematic review of the evidence regarding the effectiveness of valerian in the treatment of anxiety concluded that further, larger RCTs were needed.

Safety: Valeriana officinalis is believed to be safe, but some other species of valerian may cause liver problems. Occasional side effects include drowsiness, mild headaches and nausea. Very rarely, there may be nervousness and excitability. Pregnant or breastfeeding women shouldn't take valerian, as there is a lack of information regarding safety. If you are taking any medications, speak to your GP or pharmacist first before using it – it can cause delirium when taken alongside loperamide, a drug used to treat diarrhoea, and the SSRI antidepressant fluoxetine.

Available as: tablets (e.g. Stressless and Kalms), a liquid extract (e.g. ESI Passiflora and Valerian Plus) and a tincture (e.g. Dormeasan).

Vervain

What it is: vervain is a perennial plant with lilac flowers. Both the leaf and flower are used in herbal medicine.

Beneficial effects: it relieves nervous tension and depression and induces sound sleep.

How it works: vervain's active ingredients include tannins and glycosides (plant sugars), but it is not known how these work.

Evidence of effectiveness: vervain has long been used as a nerve soother and to promote sound sleep, but there is no clinical evidence to support its use.

Safety: vervain may induce contractions, so it is not recommended during pregnancy.

Available as: tablet form (e.g. Stressless).

Vitamin B complex

What it is: vitamin B complex is a group of vitamins with various important roles in the body, including within the nervous system. You may be short of B vitamins if you eat a lot of processed foods, if you are a vegan, or if you are under a lot of stress.

Beneficial effects: vitamin B complex eases anxiety symptoms, including panic attacks and OCD, and depression, and promotes sound sleep.

How it works: B vitamins are involved in various processes affecting the nervous system, including the production of the neurotransmitters serotonin and GABA, and maintaining a steady supply of glucose to the brain.

Evidence of effectiveness: research suggests that vitamin B supplementation may be helpful for people suffering from depression and anxiety; several studies demonstrate a link between low levels of thiamine (vitamin B1) and anxiety, and suggest that vitamin B supplements improve symptoms. A review at the University of Oxford in 2004 of three RCTs investigating the effectiveness of folic acid (vitamin B3) concluded it may have a role in the treatment of depression. Research shows that vitamin B6 relieves PMS symptoms, such as irritability, tiredness and depression. A review of studies examining the link between low intakes of folic acid and vitamin B12 and depression recommended supplementation of these vitamins for this condition. Research published in the *Journal of Clinical Psychopharmacology* in 2001 reported that supplementing the diet with vitamin B8 (inositol) may help relieve both panic attacks and OCD. All of the B vitamins are involved in the production of serotonin, which the body uses to make the sleep-inducing hormone melatonin.

Safety: taking B vitamins is generally safe; however you should take a supplement containing no more than 100 mg of vitamin B6, as higher doses can cause nerve damage. If you are pregnant or breastfeeding, suffer from gout, diabetes, or liver problems, or have had a stomach ulcer, speak to your GP or pharmacist before taking a vitamin B complex supplement.

Available as: tablets (e.g. Solgar B-Complex with Vitamin C Stress Formula) and capsules.

Herb/Supplement Selector

Use this checklist to help you select the right herb/supplement for you.

Condition	Herb(s)	Supplement(s)
Anxiety	Californian poppy, camomile, hawthorn, lemon balm, passion flower, Rhodiola rosea, skullcap	GABA, 5-HTP, fish/flax oil, magnesium, vitamin B complex
Anxiety with insomnia	Camomile, hops, lemon balm, passion flower, skullcap, valerian, vervain	GABA, 5-HTP, magnesium, vitamin B complex
Depression	St John's wort	5-HTP, fish/flax oil, cod liver oil, flaxseed oil, SAMe, vitamin B complex
Seasonal affective disorder (SAD)	St John's wort	5-HTP
Panic attacks		5-HTP, vitamin B complex
Phobias		GABA, 5-HTP
Obsessive compulsive disorder (OCD)	St John's wort	5-HTP, vitamin B complex
Body dysmorphic disorder	St John's wort	5-HTP

Review the benefits

To decide whether it is worth continuing to take a supplement, review the benefits it has on your anxiety symptoms. Evaluate your anxiety symptoms on a scale of zero to ten before you start using the supplement, and then repeat after three months of use.

Chapter 4

Get Active

Another possible factor in the rising levels of anxiety disorders in the UK is people's increasingly sedentary lifestyles. The rise in car ownership and use of public transport means fewer people walk or cycle on a daily basis and – along with our increased use of labour-saving domestic appliances and more of us than ever working in office jobs – means we are far less active than previous generations.

Research suggests that being physically active can help both prevent and ease anxiety; exercise uses up the 'fight or flight' hormones adrenaline and cortisol that are released during the stress response. Also, during exercise, the body releases the 'happy' hormone serotonin and endorphins that act as natural tranquillisers, reducing anxiety and stress, and boosting mood. A study in the Netherlands in 2006 looked at how regular exercise affected levels of anxiety and depression. Over 19,000 teenage- and adult-twins and their families took part. The researchers concluded that the participants who exercised regularly were less likely to suffer from anxiety and depression than those who were less active. Another RCT in the Netherlands in 2002 suggested that exercise may be effective in treating panic attacks.

Studies also suggest that people who take regular exercise have higher self-esteem – possibly because they feel better about their body image and feel a sense of achievement after exercising. Attending an exercise class or a gym is also a good way to meet other people with common interests, which can also have a beneficial effect on mental health.

However, you don't necessarily have to go to the gym to become more active. This chapter also looks at ways of fitting exercise into your everyday routine. Activities such as walking, housework, outdoor exercise, Pilates, swimming, t'ai chi and yoga, and the mental health benefits they offer, are discussed.

18 Walk more

Walking is a great way to improve your mental health and general fitness. An eight-year study in the US showed that menopausal women who walked for 40 minutes at least five times a week experienced less stress, anxiety and depression than less active women. Even if you are very busy, it is possible to fit more walking into your daily routine. There are the obvious strategies, such as parking your car further from the office or the shops, or getting off the bus or train one stop earlier, but other easy ways to walk more include:

- Park your car at the top of a multi-storey car park, then use the stairs down and back up.

- Get up from your desk and walk around regularly.

- Use the stairs instead of the lift.

- Take a 15-minute walk during your lunch break, instead of sitting at your desk.

- Walk to your colleagues' desks to pass on information rather than emailing them.

- Walk to the water dispenser every hour for a refill – your mind will benefit from the exercise and the increased hydration.

- Make trips to the kitchen to make drinks for colleagues.

- Walk your dog every day – if you don't have one, offer to walk your neighbour's.

19 Be a domestic god/goddess

Doing the housework is another way of fitting physical activity into your daily routine and boosting your mental health. Vacuuming, dusting and cleaning don't just give the body a good workout; research published in the *British Journal of Sports Medicine* in 2008 suggests that it also reduces the risk of suffering from anxiety and depression. The findings were based on the responses of 20,000 people in Scotland: around 3,200 of these respondents said they suffered from anxiety or depression, and the respondents who did housework or sport regularly were the least likely to suffer. The report claimed that a 20-minute session of housework reduced the risk of depression by 20 per cent.

20 Enjoy ecotherapy

Research at Essex University, commissioned by the mental health charity Mind and published in 2007, reported that ecotherapy (engaging with nature) offers both mental and physical health benefits. In one study, 108 people took part in 'green exercise' activities, such as gardening, walking, cycling and conservation work. Of these, 94 per cent reported benefits to their mental health, such as feeling more relaxed and having improved self-esteem.

Even a passive pastime like admiring a view has been shown to reduce stress and ease muscular tension. Experts claim that the higher levels of negative ions near areas with running water, trees and mountains may play a part. Others suggest that the success of ecotherapy is down to biophilia – the theory that we all have an innate affinity with nature and that our disconnection from it is the cause of stress and mental health problems. Studies in the Netherlands and Japan have suggested that people living in or near green areas enjoy a longer and healthier life than those living in urban environments.

As a result of these findings, Mind called for ecotherapy – especially 'green exercise' – to be more widely recognised as a valid treatment for mental distress. To benefit from ecotherapy, aim to spend some time outdoors in a green space, such as a garden, park or woodland, each day. To gain the most benefit, try to incorporate some exercise such as walking, cycling or gardening. Being outdoors also gives the added benefits of exposure to sunlight, such as increased vitamin D levels and better sleep.

21 Practise Pilates

Pilates is a low-impact exercise programme devised by the gymnast Joseph H. Pilates to firm the abdominal (core) muscles and generally lengthen and strengthen all of the muscles in the body. It encourages good posture, which promotes a positive mood, as well as deep, controlled breathing, which can help alleviate stress. In her book *Pilates for Every Body*, the US fitness programme presenter Denise Austin recommends Pilates for improving your mental outlook. She says that the smooth steady movements have a quietening effect on the mind and can soothe away tension.

Pilates can be practised at home – there are various instructional DVDs available, but it is probably best to join a class initially, to ensure that you adopt the correct posture and perform the exercises properly. Most leisure centres and health clubs now offer Pilates classes. The Body Control Pilates Association provides details of qualified instructors (see Directory).

22 Get in the swim

According to the Chief Medical Officers's report *At least five a week: Evidence on the impact of physical activity and its relationship to health,* which was published in 2004, swimming has psychological as well as physical benefits. The report highlights the calming effect of swimming; many people find being in the water relaxing, probably because it supports the weight of the body. Also, when you are swimming you have to focus on your breathing, rhythm and stroke, which helps take your mind off any nagging worries. To improve your swimming technique, visit www.swimfit.com, a website that offers animated swimming stroke guides.

23 Try t'ai chi

T'ai chi, described as a moving meditation, is an ancient Chinese art that promotes both mental and physical well-being. The movements are slow and controlled, helping improve strength, flexibility, posture and balance. There is some evidence that t'ai chi can help reduce mental and emotional stress.

It is possible to learn t'ai chi at home using an instructional DVD, but it is probably better to learn how to perform the movements correctly by joining a class – for details of classes near you visit www.taichifinder.co.uk.

24 Say 'yes' to yoga

The word yoga comes from the Sanskrit word yuj, which means union. Yogic postures (asanas) and breathing exercises are designed to unite the body, mind and soul. Hatha yoga is a slow, gentle form of exercise that not only strengthens the joints and muscles and increases flexibility and mobility, but also relieves stress and anxiety and induces calm. In 2002, researchers at the Australian National University, Canberra, concluded that there was some evidence that yoga breathing exercises are beneficial for people with anxiety and depression. On a personal note, I find that my weekly one-hour yoga session leaves me feeling not only calmer, but also refreshed and revitalised. Below is a breathing exercise and some asanas that may help ease your anxiety symptoms when practised regularly.

Alternate nostril breathing (nadi shodana)

This yoga breathing exercise helps promote calm.

1. Place the index and middle fingers of your right hand in between your eyebrows.

2. Press your right nostril closed with your thumb. Inhale slowly through your left nostril.

3. Holding your breath, release your right nostril and block your left nostril with your ring finger.

4. Exhale slowly through your right nostril. Then release the left nostril and inhale.

5. Repeat this cycle five to ten times.

The tree (vrksasana)

This asana calms the mind and improves balance.

1. Stand with your feet slightly apart, your knees straight and your arms and shoulders relaxed.

2. Exhaling, place your left foot on the inside of your right thigh, as high up as you can, with the toes pointing downwards.

3. Inhaling, stretch your arms to the sides palms facing down.

4. Exhaling, join your hands together in the prayer position.

5. Raise your arms above your head keeping your hands in the prayer position. To help you keep your balance, focus on a point in front of you and keep on breathing in and out, slowly and rhythmically. Stay in the pose for about 1 minute.

6. Repeat on the other side.

Learn yoga

The best and probably the most enjoyable way to learn yoga is to attend classes run by a qualified teacher. To find one near you, go to the British Wheel of Yoga's website – www.bwy.org. uk. If you'd prefer to teach yourself at home, visit www.abc-of-yoga.com, a site which shows you how to do the various postures using animated clips. You can buy CDs and MP3 hatha yoga class downloads, suitable for all levels and abilities, and download a free 'taster session' at www.yoga2hear.co.uk. You can also find yoga information, products and guidance at www.yoga-abode.com.

Safe yoga

When practising yoga at home, always proceed gently and avoid forcing your body into postures. Stop immediately if you feel any discomfort. Wear lightweight, loose clothing, to allow you to move freely, and no footwear, as yoga is best performed barefoot. Use a non-slip mat if the floor is slippery. Don't attempt inverted postures if you have a neck or back problem, or have high blood pressure, heart disease or circulatory problems. If in doubt, consult your GP first.

Chapter 5

Stress Management

Excessive stress can trigger anxiety, and anxiety can provoke the stress response, leading to a vicious cycle of stress and worry. It's thought that stress may cause chemical changes in the brain, which result in reduced levels of neurotransmitters like calming gamma-aminobutyric acid (GABA) and mood-boosting serotonin, making us feel anxious and depressed.

This chapter explains what stress is and offers stress management and relaxation techniques to help you deal with stress better and thus reduce your anxiety levels and boost your mood.

What is stress?

Stress is basically the way the mind and body respond to situations and pressures that leave us feeling inadequate or unable to cope. One person may cope well in a situation that another might find stressful; it's all down to the individual's perception of it and ability to deal with it.

How does stress affect the body?

The brain reacts to stress by preparing the body to either stay put and face the perceived threat, or escape from it. It does this by releasing hormones – chemical messengers –including adrenaline, noradrenaline and cortisol, into the bloodstream. These speed up the heart rate and breathing patterns and can induce sweating, as glucose and fatty acid levels in the blood rise in order to provide a burst of energy to deal with the threat. This is called the 'fight or flight' response.

Nowadays, the situations that induce the stress response are unlikely to necessitate either of these reactions. Those pressures that continue for a long period of time with no end in sight, for example long-term unemployment, illness or an unhappy relationship, mean that stress hormone levels remain high, increasing blood pressure and the risk of major health conditions, such as coronary heart disease and stroke, and lowering immunity to infections. Other psychological and physical symptoms include anxiety, irritability, depression, poor concentration, headaches, skin problems, allergies, poor appetite or overeating, indigestion, IBS and palpitations, so it's important to find ways to reduce and deal with stress. According to the Health & Safety Executive, work-related stress caused workers in Great Britain to lose 11.3 million working days in 2013/14.

What can I do about stress?

There are three things you can do to manage stress: avoid it, reduce it and relieve it.

25 Keep a stress diary

Over a couple of weeks, note down the details of situations, times, places and people that make you feel stressed. Once you've identified these, think about each one and ask yourself: 'Can I avoid it?' For example, if you find driving to work during the rush hour stressful, perhaps you can avoid doing it by starting or finishing work a little earlier or later or by car-sharing with a colleague?

If you cannot avoid it, you can usually reduce the level of stress you experience by changing your attitude towards a situation, or by taking practical steps to help you cope better. You can also relieve the effects of stress by practising relaxation techniques and doing things that help you unwind.

26 Remind yourself that life is OK

As well as recognising the external factors that make you feel stressed, consider whether some aspects of your personality are also to blame. Are you a perfectionist who is never satisfied with your achievements and lifestyle? Constantly feeling that who you are and what you have aren't good enough can lead to unrealistic expectations, discontent and unnecessary pressure. In his best-selling book *Don't Sweat the Small Stuff,* the late Dr Richard Carlson urged us to remind ourselves that 'life is okay the way it is, right now'. Adopting this attitude immediately reduces stress and induces calm.

Cut down on having and concentrate on being

In his book *Affluenza*, the psychologist Oliver James warns that our preoccupation with acquiring more and more material goods means that we end up working longer and longer hours, becoming more tired, stressed and prone to anxiety. He suggests that, before buying something, you should ask yourself whether you need it or simply want it, and that when you do this you will soon realise that you are spending more than you need to. He advocates cutting down on having and concentrating on being. This is good, sound advice that also reduces the risk of becoming debt-ridden, with all of the worries that money problems can cause.

27 Remember that you'll never reach the end of your 'to-do' list

Workaholism is another factor that tends to be linked with perfectionism – a 'perfect' home and lifestyle have to be paid for. While working hard for what you want in life is commendable, some people work such long hours that they don't have time to enjoy what they have. If you're constantly driven to get everything done, and think you'll feel calm and relaxed once everything on your 'to-do' list is completed, think again! What tends to happen is that, as you complete tasks, you add new ones to your list, so you never get to the end of it. It's a fact of life that there will always be tasks to be completed.

28 Change your attitude

When difficult situations do come along, changing your attitude towards them can reduce the amount of stress they cause, because it is your interpretation of the event, not the event itself, that elicits your emotional response. When something bad happens, instead of thinking about how awful the situation is, try to find something positive about it if you can. Try to find solutions to your problems, or view them as opportunities for personal growth. For example, being made redundant initially seems like a negative event but, if you view it as an opportunity to retrain and start a new career doing something you really enjoy, it can become a catalyst for positive change.

29 Live in the moment

Research shows that living in the moment, or practising mindfulness, reduces stress levels and helps alleviate anxiety. It involves giving all of your attention to the here and now, rather than worrying about the past or future, and has its roots in Buddhism. It's based on the philosophy that you can't alter the past or foretell the future, but you can influence what's happening in your life right now. By living fully in the present, you can perform to the best of your ability, whereas worrying about the past and future can hamper how you function now, and increase your stress levels unnecessarily.

Living in this way means your experience of life is richer because, instead of doing things on autopilot, all of your senses will be fully engaged in what you are doing. Imagine going for a walk in the park while being so preoccupied with worries about the future or regrets about the past that you don't even notice your surroundings. Then think how much more pleasurable and relaxing the experience would be if you took the time to absorb the sights, sounds and smells around you. When you focus on the here and now, you will find yourself appreciating the simple things in your life more.

In his book *Stop Thinking, Start Living*, Dr Richard Carlson suggested that anxiety and depression are the result of dwelling on the past or thinking about the future and that the way to healthy mental-functioning is to focus your attention on the present. He said that living in the present means that you will always do the best you can at the time and, when problems arise, you will take appropriate action. As you focus your energies on what you can do in the present time to solve a problem, it will no longer seem insurmountable.

I have also found that living in the present means that I concentrate on dealing with actual problems, instead of worrying about ones that haven't happened yet – and may never happen. This automatically reduces my anxiety levels.

Dr Carlson also claimed that problems become easier to solve when you focus on what actions you can take now to resolve them. Even taking the tiniest step towards a solution can make you feel better and more in control of your situation, which in turn reduces stress levels. You can develop your ability to focus on the present by practising simple meditation, which is discussed a little further on in this chapter.

Mindfulness is also about being happy with your life as it is now, rather than wishing things were different. Octavius Black, co-author of *The Mind Gym: Give Me Time*, suggests that we should 'make today be tomorrow's happy memories'. Adopting this attitude towards life will immediately lower your stress levels. If you find it hard to focus on the present, try keeping a daily diary. For more information on mindfulness and for a mindfulness exercise, take a look at the Mental Health Foundation's Be Mindful campaign (see Directory).

Try not to worry about 'what ifs'

Worrying about events that haven't even happened can bring on the stress response, as your body can't differentiate between what has actually happened and what you imagine happening.

For example, if you fear that you might be made redundant and will be unable to pay your mortgage, your body will produce stress hormones, even if you don't actually lose your job. Although it's hard not to worry about the things that might go wrong in your life, it's better for your mental health if you can make a conscious decision not to worry about things that haven't happened yet.

30 Simplify your life

If you feel that your life is spiralling out of control, with too many demands from your work, home, partner, family and friends, maybe it's time to simplify your life. If you regularly feel under pressure and stressed because of a lack of time, try reviewing how you structure your days. Keep a diary for a week to see how you spend your time and then decide which activities you can cut out or reduce to make more time for the things that are most important to you. Try saying 'no' to the non-essential tasks you don't have time for, or just don't want to do. It's a little word, but it can dramatically reduce your stress levels. If you find it hard to say 'no', then perhaps you need to develop your assertiveness skills.

Slow down

Many of us are living our lives at a faster and faster pace, perhaps juggling a full-time job with a relationship, family commitments and a social life. As a result, we feel a constant sense of urgency in our daily lives as we race from one task to another. This constant feeling of pressure fuels our impatience when we have to wait in a queue or traffic jam, or when the bus or train is late. Octavius Black says that we need to accept that we will never have enough time to do everything. He believes that, in order to enjoy the moment, we need to slow down, perhaps viewing situations such as queuing or travel delays as welcome thinking or reading time, rather than allowing impatience and frustration to raise our levels of stress and anxiety unnecessarily.

Prioritise
When you have a long 'to-do' list, number tasks in terms of urgency and importance, and carry them out in that order.

Delegate
Perfectionism can also lead to a need to control – you convince yourself that no one else can meet your high standards, so you do everything yourself. This inevitably leads to physical and mental overload. The solution is to accept that you can't know and do everything, so you need to learn to listen to other people's ideas and opinions and to delegate: ask your partner and children to help with domestic tasks and accept any offers of help at work.

Clear away clutter
If a bulging wardrobe, heaving shelves and overflowing cupboards are getting you down, make your life simpler and less stressful by getting rid of unnecessary clutter around your home. You'll save time and energy, because you'll find things more quickly in a clutter-free environment and your mental clarity will improve, because ridding yourself of physical clutter is very soothing. Tidying up before you prepare for bed also helps you fall asleep more quickly, according to sleep expert Dr Beata O'Donoghue. She says that clutter raises levels of the stress hormone cortisol, which stops you from winding down. If you haven't worn, read or used an item for two years or more, give it to a charity shop, sell it on eBay, or throw it away. If you can't bear to get rid of it, store it in the loft, then make it a rule that if you haven't thought about using the item within six months, it is time to part with it. If you

have a lot of possessions to sort out, ask your partner, a family member or a friend to help you. You'll be amazed at how much happier and less stressed you will feel after a good clear-out.

31 Assert yourself

If you feel you often hide your true feelings instead of expressing them, and give in to others to gain their approval, or so that you don't hurt or upset them, you might benefit from brushing up on your assertiveness skills. People who are able to express how they feel effectively are less likely to suffer from depression and social anxiety.

Do you regularly allow others to manipulate you into doing things you don't want to do? Being assertive empowers you to say what you want, feel and need, calmly and confidently, without being aggressive or hurting others. The following techniques will help you express your emotions and remain in control of your life, doing things because you want to, rather than to please other people; being 'true to yourself' will automatically reduce your anxiety and stress levels.

- Demonstrate ownership of your thoughts, feelings and behaviour by using 'I' rather than 'we', 'you' or 'it'. Rather than saying 'You make me angry', try something like 'I feel angry when you…' This is less antagonising to the other person.

- When you have a choice whether to do something or not, say 'won't' rather than 'can't' to show that you've made an active decision, rather than suggesting that something or someone has stopped you. Say 'choose to' instead of 'have to' and 'could' rather than 'should', to indicate that you have a choice. For example: 'I won't be going out tonight', rather than 'I can't go out tonight', or 'I could go out tonight, but I have chosen to stay in'.

- When you feel that your needs aren't being considered, state what you want calmly and clearly, repeating it until the other person shows they've heard and understood what you've said.

- When making a request, identify exactly what it is you want and what you're prepared to settle for. Choose positive, assertive words, as outlined above, for example: 'I would like you to help me tidy the kitchen' or 'I'd really appreciate it if you could empty the kitchen bin'.

- When refusing a request, speak calmly but firmly, giving the reason or reasons why without apologising. Repeat if you need to. For example: 'I won't be able to babysit for you tonight because I'm feeling really tired after being at work all day.'

- When you disagree with someone, say so using the word 'I'. Explain why you disagree, but acknowledge the other person's right to have a different viewpoint. For example: 'I don't agree that the service in that restaurant is poor – our meal was only late last time we visited because it was very busy, but I can understand why you think that.'

32 Seek support

Suffering from anxiety can leave you feeling isolated and convinced that no one else understands what you are experiencing. Making contact with fellow sufferers or with trained support staff or counsellors may help you overcome these feelings. The following organisations offer the opportunity to do just that; further information and contact details can be found in the directory. However, if you feel that this type of support isn't enough to help you deal with the stresses in your life, don't be afraid to seek professional help. Your GP should be able to offer advice and possibly refer you to a counsellor.

- Anxiety Care is a charity based in east London that aims to help people recover from anxiety-related disorders using CBT (cognitive behavioural therapy). It offers an online support group, a helpline and an email enquiry service run by trained counsellors. The charity also runs support and recovery groups locally.

- Anxiety UK is a user-led charity offering information, support and understanding to people with anxiety disorders. It aims to reduce isolation among sufferers by providing a network of self-help groups across the UK, specialist helplines, an online forum, a chat room, an 'e-pals' service, live chat support, and email and letter support.

- First Steps to Freedom is a UK charity offering practical support to people with anxiety disorders. The services offered include a confidential helpline, where you can discuss your anxiety problems with trained volunteers, and a personal recovery CBT programme with telephone support.

- Mental Health Matters is a UK charity for people with mental health needs. It offers various services, including 24-hour helplines across the UK that are staffed by trained workers offering emotional support, including a person-centred assessment, to anyone who calls. Staff also recommend appropriate local and national mental health services to callers.

- Mind is a UK charity with over 180 local associations offering counselling, befriending and drop-in sessions. The Mind Infoline offers information, advice and support, and details of services near you.

- NHS Choices provides blogs and forums on medical conditions, including anxiety-related disorders. The blogs provide personal insight from sufferers, carers and medical professionals about symptoms, treatments, and on how to manage the condition. The forums enable people to request advice and share experiences and information.

- No Panic is a UK charity that offers worldwide support for sufferers of GAD, phobias, panic attacks and OCD. The services offered include a night-time anxiety crisis line, local self-help groups, a contact service enabling members to befriend fellow sufferers and telephone recovery groups for people who are unable to access local support groups.

- OCD Action is a charity offering information and support to people with OCD. The charity's website hosts a number of forums where you can share your thoughts and feelings about OCD, receive advice and learn about support groups in your area. Support groups can be run by someone who has OCD (with help from OCD Action), a carer with experience of the disorder, or a suitably qualified professional. These groups offer the opportunity to meet other people who have learned successful strategies for coping with the condition. There is also a help and information line.

- OCD-UK is a charity offering information and practical and emotional support to OCD sufferers. Services offered include a telephone information line, an email support service, facilitated support groups (independently run but supported by OCD-UK) and moderated online discussion forums.

- Patient UK Experience is a forum provided by Patient UK, a website offering health information 'as provided by GPs and nurses to patients during consultations'. You can read about others' experiences of medical conditions, including anxiety, panic attacks and phobias, as well as medications, treatments and services, and share your own.

- Rethink is a UK charity that offers information and advice on living with mental illness – including anxiety. The services offered include helplines, a network of self-help groups, an online discussion forum and a blog area where you will find members' diaries, experiences and views. If you are unable to, or don't wish to, attend local group meetings, you can receive help and support over the telephone or by email.

- Sane is a UK mental health charity offering information and support to people with mental health issues. Support services include SANEline – a helpline staffed by trained workers offering confidential support and information, as well as details of local services – and SANEmail, an online support service. There is also a discussion board.

- Social Anxiety UK is a volunteer-led organisation for people with social anxiety issues. There are 33 self-help groups across the UK offering social anxiety sufferers the chance to meet up and share their experiences. The website offers chat rooms and discussion boards.

- The Stress Management Society offers guidance on dealing with stress, including 'desk yoga' and 'desk massage' techniques you can practice at work, and a creative visualisation you can do whenever you have a few minutes to yourself.

Lend support to others

Helping others may also benefit your mental health. A review in 2008 at the University of Wales, Lampeter, of the evidence on the effects volunteering has on health found that volunteering improved self-esteem and helped reduce depression. There are probably several reasons for this: helping others takes your mind off yourself and your own problems; it also helps you feel more connected to other people and therefore less isolated. Being kind to others is also thought to trigger the release of opiates in the brain, which makes us feel happier and more positive about ourselves.

33 Laugh more

Laughter is a great stress reliever. A good belly laugh seems to reduce the stress hormones cortisol and adrenaline and raise mood-boosting serotonin levels. People who see the funny side of life appear to have a reduced risk of the health problems associated with stress. So make time to watch your favourite comedies and comedians, and be around people who make you laugh. Or, visit www.laughlab.co.uk or www.ahajokes.com whenever you feel like a good giggle!

34 Do something purely for pleasure

Spend time each day doing something purely for pleasure – whether it's having a long soak in a warm, scented bath, sitting down with a glass of wine and a good book, listening to your favourite music, or going to the cinema. Doing something you really enjoy will help take your mind off domestic and work pressures.

35 Get the exercise habit

Regular exercise is a great antidote to stress, because it enables the body to use the stress hormones whose purpose it is to provide the extra energy needed to run away from our aggressors, or to stay put and fight. It also triggers the release of endorphins, which act as antidepressants.

36 Breathe deeply

When we're stressed or anxious, our breathing tends to become shallow, or we hold our breath without realising it. Slow, deep breathing has been shown to reduce the heart rate, relax muscles and release tension. Research by Dr Daniel McIntosh at the University of Denver suggests that breathing through the nose reduces the temperature of blood travelling to the emotion centre of the brain and triggers the release of mood-boosting serotonin and dopamine.

Focusing on your breathing helps take your mind off your worries. So, the next time you're stressed or anxious, try taking control of your breathing with this simple exercise:

1. Inhale slowly through your nostrils to a count of five, allowing your stomach to expand.

2. Hold for a count of five.

3. Breathe out slowly through your nose to a count of five, while slowly flattening your stomach.

4. Repeat up to ten times.

37 Practise muscle relaxation

According to Richard Hilliard, director of the Relaxation for Living Institute (RFLI), it's impossible to have an anxious mind when your muscles are relaxed. The institute's website offers advice on relaxation and stress management. Several studies have shown that relaxation techniques, like the following one, are helpful for anxiety and depression.

1. Take a deep breath and then create tension in your face by clenching your teeth and screwing up your eyes tightly, then relax and breathe out.

2. Take a deep breath, then lift the muscles in your shoulders, tense them for a few seconds and then relax, dropping your shoulders and releasing the tension as you breathe out.

3. Take a deep breath, then clench your fists and tense the muscles in your arms, hold for a few seconds then release and breathe out.

4. Next, tense the muscles in your buttocks and your legs, including the thighs and calves, hold, and then release as you breathe out.

5. Finally, clench your toes and tense your feet, hold, and then release and breathe out.

38 Meditate

Research suggests that meditation lowers stress and reduces anxiety. There are various meditation techniques, but here is a simple one that can be practised whenever you have a few moments to yourself – even while on the bus or train!

Close your eyes and focus on your breathing. As you inhale slowly and deeply through your nose, expand your stomach, and hold for a few seconds, before drawing in your stomach, while exhaling slowly. Whenever your attention is distracted by a passing thought, return to simply observing your breathing. If you prefer, you can listen to a step-by-step mindfulness meditation at www.stressmanagement.co.uk.

39 Sleep soundly

Anxiety often affects sleep, because continuing to worry when you go to bed makes it impossible to switch off and fall asleep. If you do manage to drop off, it is common to wake up several times and lie there thinking about your concerns. Even if you don't wake up during the night, anxiety often leads to restless sleep. Insufficient or poor-quality sleep increases the stress response, resulting in a vicious cycle of stress, anxiety and insomnia.

To sleep more soundly, try the following:

- Get outdoors during the day. Exposure to daylight stops the production of melatonin, the brain chemical that promotes sleep, making it easier for your body to release it at night so that you fall asleep more easily and sleep more soundly.

- Make sure you're neither too hungry nor too full when you go to bed, as both can cause wakefulness.

- Don't drink coffee or cola after 2 p.m. because the stimulant effects of the caffeine they contain can last for hours. Although tea contains about half as much caffeine – around 50 mg per cup – it's best not to drink it near bedtime if you have difficulty sleeping. Redbush or herbal teas, which are caffeine-free, make good alternatives.

- Exercise can help you sleep more soundly, because it encourages your body temperature and metabolism to increase and then fall a few hours later, which promotes sleep. Try not to exercise later than early evening, as exercising too late at night can prevent you from sleeping because your body temperature may still be raised when you get into bed. Not taking enough exercise can cause sleep problems and restlessness. Even gentle stretching can help you sleep.

- Wind down before bedtime. Develop a regular routine in the evening that allows you to put the day to bed. This could involve watching TV, although it's probably best to avoid watching anything that could prey on your mind when you are trying to go to sleep. Other relaxing activities you could do include reading and listening to music.

- Soak in a warm bath at bedtime. Your temperature increases slightly with the warmth and then falls, helping you to drop off. The warmth can help relieve both physical and mental tension, epecially if you add relaxing essential oils such as lavender or camomile.

- Avoid drinking alcohol before bedtime; although it may relax you at first and help you fall asleep more quickly, it has a stimulant effect, causing you to wake up more often during the night. It's also a diuretic, making nocturnal trips to the toilet more likely. However, if abstinence doesn't help you sleep better, it may be worth indulging in a small glass of Cabernet Sauvignon, Merlot or Chianti – there's some evidence that these wines improve your sleep patterns because the grape skins they contain are rich in plant melatonin.

- Ensure that your bedroom is cool and dark. Your brain tries to reduce your body temperature at night to slow down your metabolism. To encourage sleep, aim for a temperature of around 16°C. Darkness stimulates the production of melatonin by the pineal gland in the brain.

- Make sure you choose the correct mattress. An easy way to check whether a mattress gives you the right support is to lie on your back and slip a hand under your lower back. There should be just enough space for your hand to fit in the gap between your back and the mattress. If there's no space, the mattress is probably too soft. A bed board beneath the mattress could help. If there's a lot of space, it's likely that it is too hard for you.

- Choose a pillow that will provide support for the neck and head and keep your spine in line with your neck. The Sleep Council advocates using a soft pillow and Sammy Margo, physiotherapist and author of *The Good Sleep Guide,* suggests it should be fairly flat, though the best pillow height for you depends on the width of your shoulders. For narrow shoulders, choose a flatter pillow; if you have broad shoulders, you may need two pillows.

- To help your brain associate the bedroom with sleep and sex only, avoid having a TV or computer in it. Watching TV or using a computer last thing at night can overstimulate your brain, making it harder for you to switch off and fall asleep. Also, both TV and computer screens emit bright light that may interfere with the production of melatonin.

- If mulling over problems or a busy schedule the next day stops you from falling asleep, try writing down your concerns or a plan for the day ahead before you go to bed.

- Problems that seem insignificant during the day can seem insurmountable in the middle of the night. You might have been asleep, but suddenly you find yourself wide awake, mulling over something that's going on in your life. Your mind goes into overdrive, trying to think of a solution, but there just doesn't seem to be one. It might help if you imagine your worries are inside a helium balloon, then visualise letting go of the balloon and watching it, and your worries, float away.

- Only go to bed when you feel really sleepy. If you can't drop off within what seems like around 20 minutes, get up and do something you find relaxing, such as reading or listening to calming music. Only return to your bed when you feel drowsy again – this helps reinforce your brain's connection between your bed and sleep.

Try complementary therapies

Various complementary therapies, including acupressure, aromatherapy, massage and reflexology, are thought to help relieve psychological stress and muscle tension. For ideas on how you can practise these therapies at home, see chapter 8.

Chapter 6

Adopt an Anti-anxiety Attitude

Cognitive behavioural therapy (CBT) is a form of psychotherapy that targets the thoughts (cognition) and behaviour that can play a part in anxiety disorders. Because there is good evidence that CBT can be effective in treating generalised anxiety disorder (GAD), depression, panic attacks, phobias, obsessive compulsive disorder (OCD) and post-traumatic stress disorder (PTSD), the National Institute of Clinical Excellence (NICE) endorses its use for these conditions.

About CBT

CBT uses a combination of both cognitive and behavioural theory. According to cognitive theory, we form certain negative beliefs about ourselves during childhood and these take root in our minds until they become automatic. Behavioural theory is based on Russian scientist Ivan Pavlov's discovery that animals learn to link certain events with reward or punishment. This led to the belief that our behaviours are learned as a response to past experiences and can be 'unlearned' or changed.

CBT links these two theories together and works on the principle that how you think affects the way you feel, how you feel affects the way you behave, and how you behave affects the way you think. For example, someone who, after failing an exam, thinks that they are stupid and a failure might feel so negative about themselves and their ability to pass the exam that they decide not to resit it. Such an action would reinforce their view that they are a failure. CBT aims to change people's behaviours by helping them replace negative or unrealistic thoughts with more positive and realistic ones. For example, if a person who has failed an exam still has confidence in their capabilities, they are more likely to feel optimistic about their prospects of passing it in the future and are more likely to successfully resit it – an action which will promote further positive thoughts about themselves.

This chapter gives you a brief overview of some of the key principles of CBT and suggests ways you can use them to help you deal with your anxiety. If you think a more formal approach might help you, you can ask your GP about CBT – it is available on a group or one-to-one basis.

The IAPT programme

Improving Access to Psychological Therapies (IAPT) is an NHS programme of talking therapy treatments which support frontline mental health services in treating anxiety disorders and depression. The NHS developed the IAPT programme in 2008 in recognition of a national shortage of cognitive behavioural therapy (CBT) practitioners.

The service aims to make it easier for people to access talking therapies by providing more trained therapists in GP surgeries. If counselling isn't available at your surgery, your GP will be able to refer you to a local counselling service for NHS treatment. If you prefer, you may be able to refer yourself, if that option is available where you live. You can find out what is available in your area by searching for psychological therapy services on the NHS Choices website.

CBT online

You can also access CBT online through the NHS, if your GP thinks it is appropriate and refers you. There are two computerised packages that NICE recommends:

- Beating the Blues is an online CBT course for people with anxiety and depression. It consists of eight 50-minute sessions (www.beatingtheblues.co.uk).
- FearFighter is an online ten-week CBT course designed to help people suffering from anxiety or a phobia (www.fearfighter.com).

Other free online CBT courses include MoodGYM, e-couch and Living Life to the Full. See Directory for more information.

The availability of Beating the Blues and FearFighter services on the NHS varies from one area to another, but you can also pay for them privately – see the directory for contact details.

40 Try cognitive behavioural therapy techniques

This section looks at the kinds of thoughts that can contribute to anxiety disorders and depression, and suggests ways you can change them.

Avoid making a mountain out of a molehill

This is where you turn a minor event into a major one in your mind and it can make you feel very anxious.

Exercise:

1. Note down a situation where you make/made a mountain out of a molehill. For example, 'I haven't heard from my friend Carol for ages; I must have done or said something to offend her. Perhaps I have also upset other people? I'm going to end up with no friends.'

2. Write down a brief description of what has actually happened. For example, 'Carol hasn't phoned me for three months.'

3. Now list all of the possible reasons why the situation has come about. For example, 'Carol might be too busy to call. Carol might be ill. Carol might be waiting for me to call her.'

4. Next, write down a more realistic description of the event. For example, 'Carol hasn't rung me, perhaps she has been too busy.'

5. Now jot down what actions you can take to deal with the situation, based on your new perception of it. For example, 'I will ring Carol tonight to ask how she is.'

Avoid 'black or white' thinking

This is where you view something as either 'good' or 'bad', without allowing for the fact that some situations fall somewhere in between. For example, failing an exam the first time you sit it is not necessarily bad – if you view it as a learning experience that helps you go on and achieve a pass at a later date, it could be perceived as a good or positive event.

Exercise:

1. Write down a brief description of a situation where you used 'black or white' thinking. Using the failed exam example, this could be: 'I failed my exam and decided I was a total failure.'

2. Write down any evidence you have that your thoughts were correct. This could be: 'I failed my exam.'

3. Write down any evidence you have that your thoughts are incorrect. This could be: 'I've passed exams in the past, therefore I'm not a failure.'

4. Finally, write down a more realistic way of thinking about the situation. This could be: 'I've failed the exam this time but I've passed exams in the past, so I am sure I can pass this one in the future. Now that I have sat it once I will be more prepared for the next time.'

Be realistic about the likelihood of bad events

If you suffer from anxiety, it's likely that you spend a lot of time worrying about things that might happen to you or the people you care about. The more time you spend thinking about bad events happening, the more likely you are to believe they will happen, and the more anxious you will become. While bad events do happen, they are usually relatively rare, so it is likely that you are overestimating the possibility of a negative event affecting you or someone you care about.

Exercise:

1. Write down a brief description of the event you are worried will happen. For example, 'I am afraid that I or a loved one will be killed in a plane crash.'

2. Find out what the probability of the event happening is. For example, the likelihood of being killed in a plane crash is one in 11 million.

3. Now write a short statement based on the facts. For example, 'Flying is a safe form of transport.' Remember that statement every time you start to worry about that situation.

Face your fears

According to CBT, facing your fears until your anxiety diminishes is the best way to overcome them. Cognitive behavioural therapists and co-authors of *Cognitive Behavioural Therapy for Dummies,* Rob Willson and Rhena Branch, use the acronym FEAR (Face Everything and Recover) to describe this approach. The technical terms for this process are 'desensitisation' or 'exposure'. The best way to do this is through managed exposure, which involves doing things step by step, gradually building up the length of time and degree to which you expose yourself to your fear. In order to benefit from this approach, you should not put yourself in a position where you feel overwhelmed with fear and take fright or, at the other end of the scale, act so cautiously that you don't give yourself the opportunity to master your fear. For example, if you are afraid of swimming in the deep end of the pool, one extreme might be challenging yourself to dive in at the deep end and the other simply sitting at the side of the pool at the deep end, dipping your toes in the water. You need to find a balance between these two extremes. Your managed exposure programme to overcome your fear of swimming in the deep end might look like this:

- Day one – starting at the shallow end and swimming next to the edge of the pool (so that you can grab the side if you need to), head towards the deep end, as far as you can without feeling too anxious or panicky.

- Day two – starting at the shallow end, close to the edge of the pool, swim a little further towards the deep end than you did on day one.

- Day three – follow the same steps as days one and two, but swim a little further.

- Day four onwards – continue to follow these steps, but during each session make an effort to swim further and further until you are swimming from one end of the pool to the other, while close to the side. Your eventual aim could be to swim down the centre of the pool from one end to the other.

Overcome obsessions

Obsessive disorders such as OCD involve behaviours that are designed to reduce fear in the short term, but actually maintain it in the long term. For example, a person who is afraid of contamination from dirt and germs washes their hands to make themselves feel better in the short term, but has to repeat the action many times each day in order to keep their fears at bay.

Here are some suggestions to help you overcome your obsessive thoughts and behaviours, using this scenario as an example:

- Learn to accept doubt and uncertainty as part of life – this would require the person who is afraid of contamination to accept that, if they stop constantly washing their hands, there are no guarantees that they won't catch a cold or a tummy bug. At first, this person would feel uncomfortable with the lack of certainty, but should eventually learn to live with their doubts without feeling anxious.

- Recognise that your obsessive thoughts are normal – this would involve the person with the fear of contamination accepting that everyone has similar concerns about dirt and germs from time to time but they don't view them as abnormal and, as such, don't pay that much attention to them.

- Recognise that your obsessive thoughts are just thoughts – this would mean the person with the fear of contamination accepting that, just because they fear contamination, it doesn't mean it will happen in reality, so they don't need to take extra steps, such as frequent handwashing, to avoid it.

Chapter 7

Medical and Other Treatments

If you follow the advice in this book regarding diet, exercise, stress management, and thought and behaviour change, you may notice a big improvement in your anxiety symptoms. However, as we saw in the two case studies at the beginning of the book, sometimes lifestyle change is not possible, or is not enough to relieve symptoms, and medication or another form of treatment is needed to help you cope, either in the short or long term. This chapter gives you an overview of some of the medications commonly used to treat anxiety, including what they are, how they work and common side effects. Other treatments, such as counselling and psychotherapy, are also discussed.

Use medications safely

Not everyone will suffer from side effects from taking medications and there may be others in addition to those listed – always read the leaflet that accompanies the medication and discuss any concerns with your pharmacist or GP before using it. You can report a suspected adverse reaction to a drug on the Medicines and Healthcare products Regulatory Agency (MHRA) website (see Directory). Always inform your GP or pharmacist if you are taking any vitamin, mineral or herbal supplements, as these may interact with medications or reduce their effectiveness.

---

41 Learn about medications and other treatments for anxiety

There are various types of medications that your GP can prescribe to help treat anxiety. The timescales for taking these medications vary.

Short-term medications

If your anxiety is severe and is affecting your everyday life, your GP may prescribe you medication on a short-term basis to help give you immediate relief from your symptoms. The types of short-term medication you may be prescribed are outlined as follows:

Benzodiazepines
What they are: a type of tranquilliser. They include diazepam (Valium), lorazepam (Ativan), chlordiazepoxide (Librium and

Tropium), alprazolam, oxazepam, temazepam, nitrazepam, flurazepam, loprazolam, lormetazepam, clobazam and clonazepam.

Used for: providing quick relief from anxiety.

How they work: they damp down brain activity by enhancing the effects of the neurotransmitter GABA.

Pros: they are very effective for the short-term relief of anxiety.

Cons: if you take benzodiazepines for longer than two to four weeks you may develop a tolerance to them – this is where your body gets used to a drug and you have to take higher doses to get the same effects. You may also become dependent on (addicted to) them.

Cautions: side effects can include drowsiness, confusion, clumsiness, memory loss, dizziness and light-headedness, so benzodiazepines can affect your ability to drive and operate machinery. Benzodiazepines shouldn't be taken with alcohol, because they enhance its effects. You should not stop taking the tablets suddenly, as this can cause withdrawal symptoms, including anxiety, panic attacks, feelings of unreality and, very rarely, mental breakdown. To minimise withdrawal symptoms, reduce the dose gradually over several weeks or months before finally stopping taking the drug. Your GP can advise you on how to do this.

Beta blockers

What they are: medications normally used to treat angina and high blood pressure but which can also help ease some of the physical symptoms of anxiety. They are thought to work best for short-lived symptoms. There are many different types, including acebutolol, atenolol, betaxolol, bisoprolol and carvedilol.

Used for: easing the physical symptoms of anxiety such as shaking, sweating and an increased heart rate.

How they work: they work by blocking the release of chemicals that cause these symptoms.

Pros: most people have few or mild side effects while taking beta blockers.

Cons: some people suffer from tiredness, depression, impotence and sleep problems, including vivid dreams or nightmares. Beta blockers may also increase the risk of developing Type 2 diabetes in some people.

Cautions: you should not take beta blockers if you have asthma. If you suffer from diabetes you should bear in mind that beta blockers can mask the warning signs of a low blood sugar level (hypo).

Buspirone

What it is: a medication used to treat anxiety. It is also known as BuSpar.

Used for: relieving anxiety, including physical symptoms, such as palpitations (where your heart beats more quickly than usual).

How it works: buspirone is thought to mimic the effects of serotonin in the brain.

Pros: buspirone is not thought to be addictive, but it is still used on a fairly short-term basis for anxiety.

Cons: takes about four weeks to work. Possible side effects include drowsiness, headache, dizziness, light-headedness, dry mouth, sweating, nervousness, excitement and confusion.

Cautions: speak to your GP or pharmacist before taking buspirone if you are pregnant, breastfeeding or trying to conceive, if you suffer from kidney or liver problems, or have epilepsy. Avoid drinking large amounts of grapefruit juice while taking this medication, as it can increase its effects and the risk of side effects.

Hydroxyzine

What it is: an antihistamine, which is a type of drug normally used to prevent allergic reactions. However, hydroxyzine has been shown to be effective for anxiety. Brand names include Atarax and Ucerax.

Used for: calming you down and making you feel less anxious.

How it works: hydroxyzine blocks the effects of histamine in the brain and induces calm. Also, like benzodiazepines, it slows down brain activity by helping the neurotransmitter GABA to work better.

Pros: hydroxyzine is not addictive.

Cons: it is only effective when taken over a short period of time. Side effects include drowsiness, dizziness, headache, blurred vision and dry mouth.

Cautions: speak to your GP before taking this drug if you are pregnant or breastfeeding, suffer from kidney, liver or prostate problems, have difficulty urinating, or suffer from epilepsy, the blood disorder porphyria or glaucoma.

Long-term medications

Some people with anxiety may need longer-term treatment to help them manage their anxiety. The types of longer-term medication that your GP may prescribe are as follows:

Pregabalin (Lyrica)

What it is: an antiepileptic drug.

Used for: anxiety disorder, nerve pain and epilepsy.

How it works: it reduces the release of a neurotransmitter called glutamate, which is thought to be involved in anxiety disorder.

Pros: less likely to cause nausea than SSRIs and SNRIs (see following).

Cons: common side effects include dizziness, tiredness, confusion blurred or double vision, headache, dry mouth, constipation or diarrhoea, increased appetite and weight gain. It may also cause skin reactions, such as a rash, itching or peeling.

Cautions: there is a small risk that pregabalin may worsen suicidal thoughts and behaviour – seek medical help if you are affected. Some people experience withdrawal symptoms, such as insomnia, headache, nausea, diarrhoea, flu syndrome, nervousness, depression, pain, sweating and dizziness, after stopping this medication.

Selective serotonin reuptake inhibitors (SSRIs)

What they are: antidepressants commonly used to treat depression, but which also help relieve anxiety disorders. Examples of SSRIs include fluoxetine (Prozac), paroxetine (Seroxat), citalopram (Cipramil and Paxoran), escitalopram (Cipralex), fluvoxamine (Faverin) and sertraline (Lustral).

Used for: relieving anxiety, with or without depression, as well as panic attacks, social anxiety disorder (SAD) and other phobias, such as PMS, PTSD and OCD.

How they work: they increase levels of serotonin in the brain.

Pros: SSRIs are not addictive and have a lower risk of side effects than older antidepressants (e.g. tricyclics – see following).

Cons: possible side effects include nausea, low libido, blurred vision, diarrhoea or constipation, dizziness, dry mouth, loss of appetite, sweating, agitation and insomnia.

Cautions: SSRIs should not be taken by anyone with a history of mania. Speak to your GP or pharmacist before taking SSRIs if you are pregnant or breastfeeding, or if you suffer from heart disease, diabetes, liver or kidney problems, glaucoma or epilepsy. SSRIs can interact with other drugs – especially with other antidepressants and anticlotting drugs, such as aspirin. SSRIs may increase the risk of suicidal thoughts in some people. They should be stopped gradually to avoid withdrawal symptoms.

Serotonin and noradrenaline reuptake inhibitors (SNRIs)

What they are: a type of antidepressant that includes venlafaxine (Effexor) and duloxetine (Cymbalta).

Used for: treating anxiety, OCD or depression that has not responded to SSRIs.

How they work: they increase levels of both serotonin and noradrenaline in the brain to boost alertness and improve mood by preventing their reabsorption into the nerve cells.

Pros: SNRIs are not addictive.

Cons: common side effects include nausea, constipation, diarrhoea, lack of appetite, dry mouth, blurred vision, dizziness, insomnia and sweating.

Cautions: you should not take SNRIs if you have untreated high blood pressure (hypertension), have recently had a heart attack or have an arrhythmia (irregular heart beat). Speak to your GP if you have suicidal thoughts or develop a rash while taking this medication. Speak to your GP or pharmacist before taking this medication if you are pregnant or breastfeeding or trying to conceive, if you suffer from heart, kidney or liver problems, high blood pressure, glaucoma or epilepsy, or if you or any family member has experienced mania (high mood).

Tricyclic antidepressants (TCAs)

What they are: a type of antidepressant that includes imipramine, amitriptyline, doxepin, mianserin, trazodone and lofepramine.

Used for: panic attacks, OCD and symptoms of depression, including anxiety – especially when it is linked to insomnia.

How they work: they increase levels of various neurotransmitters in the brain by preventing their reuptake.

Pros: TCAs are not thought to be addictive.

Cons: TCAs are linked to more side effects than the newer SSRIs. These include dizziness, drowsiness, slowed reaction times, confusion, visual disturbances, tremors and an irregular heartbeat. If you experience drowsiness or slowed reaction times, you shouldn't drive or operate machinery.

Cautions: an overdose can be fatal, which is one of the reasons why SSRIs are prescribed more often than TCAs. When finishing a course of TCAs, the dose needs to be tapered off gradually, to avoid withdrawal symptoms, such as dizziness, anxiety, agitation, mood swings, low mood, sleep problems, flu-like symptoms, pins and needles, diarrhoea, abdominal cramps and nausea.

Talking therapies

If your anxiety symptoms persist, your GP may also refer you to a counsellor or a psychotherapist. Many voluntary organisations offer talking therapies, as well as group support.

Counselling

Counselling is usually a short-term treatment (less than six months) that is suitable for people who have a specific problem they want to deal with, or who are experiencing difficulties in dealing with a stressful event, such as divorce or bereavement. Counselling gives you the opportunity to talk about what is troubling you and to explore any difficult feelings you are experiencing in a safe, confidential environment. A counsellor doesn't normally offer advice, but instead helps you gain a better understanding of yourself, your feelings and behaviour, as well as develop your self-esteem and your ability to take control of your own life.

There are two main types of counselling: directive – where the counsellor determines the structure of sessions – and non-directive – where you determine what is discussed.

Directive counselling

Directive forms of counselling include cognitive behavioural therapy (CBT) and Gestalt counselling. In CBT counselling, the client is encouraged to change their beliefs and behaviours by recognising negative thought patterns and replacing them with more realistic and positive ones. The counsellor may give the client 'homework', such as keeping a diary of their thoughts and feelings. Gestalt counselling focuses on the client's thought, feeling and activity patterns and promotes self-awareness. The client develops self-awareness by learning how to analyse their own behaviour and body language, as well as express any feelings they have repressed. Sessions can include 'acting out' difficult scenarios and conversations and recalling dreams.

Non-directive counselling

Non-directive forms include psychodynamic and person-centred counselling. Psychodynamic counselling is based on the theory that past events affect what we feel and experience in the present. Various methods are used to assist the client to come to terms with the past, which helps them resolve issues in the present. For example, a person who has a fear of dogs (cynophobia) may have been bitten by one during their childhood; the counsellor will help the person acknowledge and understand their fear, deal with it, and move on.

In person-centred counselling, the counsellor offers empathy, positive feedback, honesty and openness to help the client heal and make changes in their lives.

Psychotherapy

Psychotherapy may be recommended if you have long-term anxiety issues that don't appear to be linked to a specific event in your life and may be linked to more deep-rooted emotional problems. There seems to be less of a distinction between counselling and psychotherapy than in the past although, in general, counsellors tend to undergo shorter training than psychotherapists. As with counselling, psychotherapy tends to be based on particular theories such as cognitive behavioural therapy or psychodynamic therapy. However, it tends to go on for longer than counselling – usually for several months or more – and is more intensive; psychotherapists usually focus on deeply entrenched thought patterns that may have stemmed from childhood.

Referral to a mental health specialist

If your anxiety doesn't improve with medication or talking treatments, your GP may refer you to a mental health specialist, such as a clinical psychologist or a psychiatrist, who will be able to reassess your condition and devise a treatment plan for you.

Chapter 8

DIY Complementary Therapies

The main difference between complementary therapies (also known as alternative, natural or holistic therapies) and conventional Western medicine is that the former approach focuses on treating the individual as a whole, whereas the latter is symptom-led. Complementary practitioners view illness as a sign that physical and mental well-being have been disrupted, and they attempt to restore good health by stimulating the body's own self-healing and self-regulating abilities. They claim that total well-being can be achieved when the mind and body are in a state of balance, called homeostasis. Homeostasis is achieved by following the type of lifestyle advocated in this book, i.e. a healthy diet with plenty of fresh air, exercise, sleep and relaxation, combined with stress management and a positive mental attitude.

Whether complementary therapies work or not remains under debate. Some argue that any benefits are due to the placebo effect. This is where a treatment brings about improvements simply because the person using it expects it to, rather than because it has any real effect. However, it could be argued that, unlike drug treatments, which are comparatively recent, complementary therapies, such as aromatherapy, massage and reflexology, have stood the test of time, having been used to treat ailments and promote well-being for thousands of years.

The mental health charity Mind acknowledges that complementary therapies, such as those covered in this chapter, can enable people to deal with their anxiety symptoms by helping them relax and sleep better. It also states that many people with depression have found therapies such as acupuncture, massage and homeopathy helpful.

This chapter offers a brief overview and evaluation of complementary therapies that may reduce anxiety and boost mood – including acupressure and aromatherapy, Bach flower remedies, homeopathy, massage and reflexology – and includes techniques and treatments you can try for yourself.

42 Apply acupressure

Acupressure is part of traditional Chinese medicine and is often described as 'acupuncture without needles', as it works on the same points on the body. Acupuncture also resembles acupressure in that it, too, is based on the idea that life energy, or qi, flows through channels in the body known as meridians. An even passage of qi throughout the body is viewed as vital to good health. Disruption of the flow of qi in a meridian can lead to illness at any point within it. The flow of qi can be affected by various factors, including stress, emotional distress, diet and environment.

Qi is most concentrated at points along the meridians known as acupoints. There is some scientific evidence that stimulating particular acupoints can relieve pain. Using the fingers and thumbs to apply firm but gentle pressure to these points stimulates the body's natural self-healing abilities by relieving muscular tension and boosting circulation, thereby promoting good health. The application of pressure also seems to stimulate the production of endorphins and encephalins (pain-relieving hormones). Many Chinese people use acupressure to self-treat a range of common conditions. You can try the following simple acupressure techniques for yourself:

Bend pool
Also called *Quchi*, this acupoint can be found on the inside of each forearm, at the end of the elbow crease, when the arm is bent. Use the left thumb to apply pressure to this point on the right arm for a few moments and then repeat, using the right thumb on the left arm. Stimulating these points is thought to relieve anxiety.

Inner gate
Also known as *Nei Kuan*, this acupoint is positioned on the forearms, about 5 cm down from the first wrist crease and in line with the ring finger. Applying pressure here is said to relieve anxiety.

Spirit gate
Also known as *Shenmen*, this acupoint is located on the little finger side of the forearm at the crease of the wrist. Applying firm pressure to this area is believed to relieve anxiety, fear, nervousness and emotional imbalances.

Seal hall

Also known as *Yintang*, this acupoint is situated between the eyebrows, in the indentation where the bridge of the nose joins the forehead. Using both index fingers to apply firm pressure to this area for up to 2 minutes is claimed to relieve nervousness and induce calm.

Sea of tranquillity

Also known as *Shanchung*, this acupoint can be found in the middle of the breastbone, three thumb-widths up from the bottom of the bone. Applying pressure to this area using both index fingers is believed to relieve nervousness, anxiety, depression, hysteria and other emotional imbalances.

43 Use aroma power

Essential oils are extracted from the petals, leaves, stalk, roots, seeds, nuts and even the bark of plants using various methods. Aromatherapy is based on the belief that when scents released from essential oils are inhaled, they affect the hypothalamus. This is the part of the brain that governs the glands and hormones, altering mood and lowering stress and anxiety. When used in massage, baths and compresses, the oils are also absorbed through the bloodstream and transported to the organs and glands, which benefit from their healing effects.

Massage oil

In massage, you can generally use a 2-per-cent dilution: this equates to two drops per teaspoon of carrier oil. Stronger oils may need more dilution – this is mentioned where necessary in the text. A carrier oil can be any vegetable oil, including good-quality olive oil or sunflower oil, from your kitchen. Almond, sesame seed, or grapeseed oils are equally good. Never apply aromatherapy oils to broken skin. Buy the best-quality oils you can afford; like most things, you get what you pay for, and cheaper oils may not be as pure as more expensive ones. If you have sensitive skin, it may be a good idea to do a patch test before using an essential oil you haven't used before. Dab a few drops of diluted oil inside a wrist or an elbow. If there is no reaction within 24 hours, it should be safe to go ahead and use the oil.

Bergamot boost

Bergamot has a citrusy aroma that is uplifting, yet at the same time relaxing and soothing. Use it for massage or add it to the bath diluted in a carrier oil to relieve tension and anxiety.

Caution: use bergamot in no more than a 1-per-cent dilution – in higher strengths it can increase the skin's sensitivity to sunlight, making it more likely to burn.

Camomile calm

Try Roman camomile oil, either for massage or in the bath, to soothe and calm, and aid restful sleep. Alternatively, drinking camomile tea provides similar benefits.

Clary sage soother

According to Patricia Davies, author of *Aromatherapy: An A–Z*, clary sage is one of the strongest relaxants known to aromatherapists and is especially helpful for anxiety caused by the stresses of modern living. It eases tensions and relaxes tight muscles.

Patricia Davies warns that you shouldn't drink alcohol after using clary sage, as the two combined may cause nightmares.

Feel-good frankincense

Frankincense is another calming oil. It has a spicy, woody aroma and is especially recommended where anxiety brings on an asthma attack, as it is thought to slow down and deepen breathing patterns and induce a trance-like feeling. However, Patricia Davies says that asthma sufferers should use it in massage rather than in steam inhalations, as such inhalations may bring on an attack in some people.

Lavender relaxer

For speedy stress relief, sniff lavender. It contains linalool, which is thought to stimulate brain receptors for GABA, a brain chemical that induces calm. Japanese researchers reported recently that inhaling lavender oil for 5 minutes daily dramatically reduces levels of the stress hormone cortisol. You can also take lavender flowers as an infusion or tincture – a small study in 2003 suggested that lavender tincture boosted the effects of the antidepressant imipramine.

Stress-relief neroli

Neroli has a floral, citrusy smell and gentle sedative properties, making it useful for reducing short-term anxiety – e.g. before an exam or job interview. It is also effective for long-term anxiety, especially when it is linked with insomnia. Try it diluted in a carrier oil for massage, or added to the bath.

Take an aromatic bath

Fill the bath with comfortably hot water. When you are ready to get in, add six drops of essential oil (unless otherwise stated). Agitate the water with your hand to disperse the oil, which will form a thin film on the water. The warmth of the water both aids absorption through the skin and releases aromatic vapour, which is then inhaled.

44 Massage away stress

Massage involves touch – which can help reduce stress and tension, as well as physical pain. It's thought to work by stimulating the release of serotonin (a brain chemical involved in relaxation) and endorphins (the body's own painkillers). It also decreases the level of stress hormones in the blood. A review of the effectiveness of complementary therapies in the treatment of depression in 2002 at the Australian National University, Canberra, concluded that there was some evidence that massage was beneficial.

Friction – using your thumbs, apply even pressure to static points, or make small circles on either side of the spine.

Hacking – relax your hands, then, using the sides, alternately deliver short, sharp taps all over.

Kneading – using alternate hands, squeeze and release flesh between the fingers and thumbs, as though you're kneading dough.

Stroking/effleurage – glide both hands over the skin in rhythmic fanning or circular motions.

Playing some relaxing music in the background can help enhance the feelings of relaxation; a study in 2008 involving 236 pregnant women reported that listening to classical music helped relieve stress, anxiety and depression during pregnancy.

45 Try the Emotional Freedom Technique (EFT)

Like acupuncture and acupressure, the Emotional Freedom Technique (EFT) is an energy therapy based on meridian theory. According to EFT, many of us suppress negative emotions, which are then stored in the meridians where they disrupt the flow of energy and cause more negative feelings. The technique is derived from the Chinese system of chi kung, which involves tapping on particular points to rebalance the energy flow throughout the body. In EFT, you repeat a statement that describes your negative emotions in a way that makes you feel more positive, while tapping particular points on your meridians. This is thought to send a pulse of energy through the meridians and dispel negative emotions. A similar technique, called thought field therapy (TFT), has been adapted and used by the hypnotherapist Paul McKenna to help people overcome psychological problems, such as stress, anxiety and food cravings.

Reduce panic and fear

First of all, put your fear into words, for example, 'I am terrified of spiders.' Next, to help you feel more positive about yourself, add the words, 'Even though […], I deeply love and approve of myself', so that the statement becomes: 'Even though I am terrified of spiders, I deeply love and approve of myself.'

Next, using the tips of your index and middle fingers tap five times on the 'under nose' meridian point, situated between your nose and your top lip. As you do so, repeat your statement, so that you focus on the fear you want to tackle.

Reduce anxiety and increase confidence

Put your anxiety into words, for example, 'I am worried about meeting new people.' Then reframe it with the words, 'Even though […], I deeply love and approve of myself', so that the statement becomes: 'Even though I am worried about meeting new people, I deeply love and approve of myself.'

Next, using your right index and middle fingers, tap five times on the meridian point situated on the side of your left hand, below the little finger, repeating your statement to help you focus on the worry you want to eradicate. Repeat on the other hand.

46 Use flower power

Flower essences have been used for their healing properties for thousands of years. However, it was Dr Edward Bach, a Harley Street doctor, bacteriologist and homeopath, who developed their use in the twentieth century. He believed that negative emotions were the root cause of disease and he identified 38 basic negative states of mind and devised a plant- or flower-based remedy for each. The remedies are thought to help counteract negative emotions, such as fear, despair and uncertainty, but there's only anecdotal evidence regarding their effectiveness.

The remedies are made by infusing flower heads in spring water in direct sunlight, or by boiling twigs from trees, bushes or plants. The infusion is then mixed with brandy (to act as a preservative) to make a tincture. The remedies can be taken diluted in water, or you can apply them neat to your lips, temples, wrists or behind your ears. They're widely available in pharmacies in 10-ml and 20-ml phials. The following list of Bach remedies may be helpful for anxiety and anxiety-related disorders:

- Aspen – for when you feel nervous and anxious but don't know why.

- Centaury – for excessive anxiety and an inability to say 'no'.

- Gorse – for feelings of hopelessness and despair.

- Mimulus – for irrational fears (phobias), such as a fear of flying or of spiders.

- Mustard – for melancholy.

- Red Chestnut – for overanxiety and concern for others.

- Rescue Remedy – combines five remedies, including cherry plum, rock rose and clematis, and is designed to help you cope during times of acute stress, such as exams, bereavement, etc. This remedy is also available as a handy oral spray.

- Rock Rose – for when you are 'frozen with fear'.

- Scleranthus – for mood swings.

- White Chestnut – for unwanted thoughts, worries and preoccupations.

For further information on how to select a suitable flower remedy and an online questionnaire that enables you to select a personalised blend, visit www.bachfloweressences.co.uk.

47 Get help with homeopathy

Homeopathy means 'same suffering' and is based on the idea that 'like cures like' – substances that can cause symptoms in a well person can treat the same symptoms in a person who is ill. For example, coffee contains caffeine – excessive amounts of caffeine can cause nervousness and overexcitement, so the remedy Coffea is often prescribed for these very symptoms (see the following list of remedies).

Symptoms such as inflammation or fever are viewed as a sign that the body is trying to heal itself. The theory is that homeopathic remedies encourage this self-healing process and that they work in a similar way to vaccines.

The substances used in homeopathic remedies come from plant, animal, mineral, bark and metal sources. These substances are turned into a tincture, which is then diluted many times over. Homeopaths claim that the more diluted a remedy is, the higher its potency and the lower its potential side effects. They believe in the 'memory of water': the theory that even though the molecules from a substance are diluted they leave behind an electromagnetic 'footprint' – like a recording on an audiotape – which has an effect on the body.

These ideas are controversial and many GPs remain sceptical. Evidence to support homeopathy exists, but critics argue that much of it is inconclusive. For example, research published in 2005 reported improvements in symptoms and well-being among 70 per cent of patients receiving individualised homeopathy. The study involved 6,500 patients over a six-year period at the Bristol Homeopathic Hospital. Critics of the studies argue there was no comparison group and patients may have given a positive response because it was expected. A review of eight randomised controlled trials (RCTs) of the use of homeopathy for GAD and other types of anxiety, at the University of Westminster in 2006, concluded that there was limited evidence of any benefit. This was because the results were contradictory or failed to provide enough information about the methods used. The review also reported that several uncontrolled trials had positive results, but the evidence was deemed inconclusive, owing to the lack of a controlled group. The reviewers recommended that further, more robust research should be done. However, surveys suggest that people with anxiety often use homeopathy, so it may well be worth trying.

There are two main types of remedies – whole person-based and symptom-based. It's probably best to consult a qualified homeopath who will prescribe a remedy aimed at you, as a whole person and based on your personality, as well as the symptoms you experience. However, if you prefer, you can buy homeopathic remedies at many high-street pharmacies and health shops.

The following is a list of homeopathic remedies, along with the anxiety-related physical and psychological symptoms for which they're commonly recommended. To self-prescribe, simply choose the remedy with indications that most closely match your symptoms. Follow the dosage instructions on the product.

Aconite
Physical symptoms: chest pains.
Psychological symptoms: fear, shock and anxiety; panic attacks; social phobia.

Arsen alb
Physical symptoms: restlessness and exhaustion.
Psychological symptoms: persistent anxiety; insecurity.

Aurum
Physical symptoms: headaches; palpitations.
Psychological symptoms: feelings of worthlessness and fear of failure.

Avena sativa (oats)
Physical symptoms: exhaustion.
Psychological symptoms: anxiety; inability to concentrate; nervous exhaustion and insomnia.

Calc carb
Physical symptoms: fatigue.
Psychological symptoms: insomnia; irrational fears; agoraphobia (fear of open spaces) or acrophobia (fear of heights).

Coffea
Physical symptoms: restlessness; headaches; palpitations.
Psychological symptoms: nervousness and overexcitement.

Gelsemium
Physical symptoms: weakness and shakiness.
Psychological symptoms: fear of future events and of appearing in public.

Phosphorous
Physical symptoms: palpitations.
Psychological symptoms: oversensitivity and needing reassurance; fear of the dark and of thunderstorms; fears that develop into phobias after too much solitude.

Sepia

Physical symptoms: exhaustion.

Psychological symptoms: irritability and oversensitivity; anxiety that is worse in the evening.

Not a quick fix

Practitioners warn that homeopathy isn't a 'quick fix' – the remedies may take a while to take effect. Homeopathic remedies are generally considered safe and don't have any known side effects, though sometimes a temporary worsening of symptoms, known as aggravation, may take place. This is seen as a good sign, as it suggests that the remedy is encouraging the healing process. If this happens, stop taking the remedy and wait for your symptoms to improve. If there is steady improvement, don't restart the remedy. If the improvement stops, resume taking the remedy.

---

48 Find relief in reflexology

Reflexology is based on the idea that points on the feet, hands and face, known as reflexes, correspond to different parts of the body, e.g. glands and organs. These are linked via vertical zones, along which energy flows. Illness occurs when these zones become blocked. Stimulating the reflexes using the fingers and thumbs is thought to bring about physiological changes which remove these blockages and encourage the mind and body to self-heal.

Practitioners believe that imbalances in the body result in granular deposits in the relevant reflex, which cause tenderness.

Corns, bunions and even hard skin are all believed to indicate problems in the related parts of the body. The energy theory behind reflexology is very similar to the one underpinning acupressure, although practitioners say it is a different system. There is no reliable evidence that reflexology relieves anxiety disorders, but there's anecdotal evidence that reflexology massage is relaxing. So, at the very least, trying these techniques may relieve stress and thus lessen the frequency of your symptoms.

A reflexologist will usually work on your feet because they believe that the feet are more sensitive. However, it's usually easier to work on your hands when you are self-treating.

According to Ann Gillander, author of *A Gaia Busy Person's Guide to Reflexology*, working on the brain and spine reflexes on the hand can help alleviate depression.

Contact the brain reflex

Using your left thumb and index finger, apply firm pressure to the tip of your thumb, then to the tip of your index finger and finally to the tip of your middle finger on your right hand. Repeat on your left hand, using your right thumb and index finger.

Contact the spine reflex

Using firm pressure, creep your left thumb along the outer edge of your upturned right palm, starting just above your wrist and ending about two-thirds of the way up your thumb.

Relieve anxiety and panic

This technique is said to relieve stress, anxiety and panic. Grip your right index finger with your left hand and squeeze firmly until you can feel your pulse, then release it. Repeat the action on your middle, ring and little fingers and then repeat on your right hand.

49 Help anxiety with self-hypnosis

A review of 14 RCTs investigating the effectiveness of hypnosis for the treatment of anxiety at Exeter and Plymouth universities in 2007 concluded that there was some 'limited but consistent evidence' that it may be of benefit.

Most people can learn safe and simple self-hypnosis techniques. The following steps will take you through a basic self-hypnosis, which could aid relaxation and positive thinking and possibly help ease your anxiety symptoms.

1. Lie or sit comfortably in a quiet place, where you're unlikely to be disturbed.

2. Focus on your breathing – breathe slowly and deeply.

3. Start counting backwards from 300. If your mind starts to drift away, simply start counting backwards again.

4. Begin relaxing each part of your body. Feel the muscles in your face relax, then those in your neck and shoulders, back, arms and legs, and finally your feet.

5. Now repeat an affirmation – a positive statement about yourself that describes how you would like to feel – as though it is already true. For example: 'I'm confident and relaxed in all situations.' When you're ready to come out of your trance, start counting to ten, telling yourself 'when I reach five I'll start to awaken, when I reach ten I'll wake up, feeling confident and relaxed'.

50 Use visualisation to overcome phobias

Visualisation involves using your imagination to create a picture of the situation you want to achieve in your mind. Using visualisation during self-hypnosis appears to improve its success and is called hypnotic imaging.

It is claimed that the more senses you use in your visualisation, the more effective it is likely to be.

Follow the self-hypnosis techniques outlined in action 49, then follow these steps:

1. Focus on the phobia you want to overcome.

2. Now imagine yourself confronting your phobia. Visualise the things you would see, hear the sounds you would hear and imagine the emotions you would feel once you have overcome your phobia. For example, a person who is afraid of swimming in deep water might picture themselves swimming in the deep end, hearing the splash of other people jumping into the water and experiencing the elation they would feel when they reach the other end of the pool.

3. Finally, imagine a more relaxed you, free from fear. Imagine what this new, relaxed you is like and feel how much better you feel when you are in a relaxed state.

Recipes

This section contains recipes based on some of the dietary recommendations outlined earlier in the book.

Banana and cinnamon porridge (serves one)

This recipe contains tryptophan-rich oats, milk and bananas, to help you relax. The milk also contains calming calcium, and the cinnamon helps keep your blood sugar levels steady.

Ingredients
25 g porridge oats
150 ml milk (semi-skimmed/full-fat)
1 banana, sliced
Ground cinnamon

Method
1. Cook the porridge according to the instructions on the packet.

2. Arrange the sliced banana over the porridge.

3. Add more milk to taste.

4. Sprinkle with cinnamon and serve.

5. For an extra warming breakfast, pop the finished dish in the microwave for 30 seconds to heat the banana and milk through.

Fruity muesli (serves one)

In this recipe, the oats, nuts, seeds and natural yoghurt balance the blood sugar and provide B vitamins, magnesium, selenium, zinc and tryptophan. The dried fruits and yoghurt are good sources of calcium and the berries contain antioxidants.

Ingredients
100 g oats
½ tsp cinnamon
25 g dried apricots, chopped
25 g raisins, or dried prunes or dates, chopped
1 tbsp Brazil nuts, chopped
1 tbsp pumpkin seeds
1 tbsp sunflower seeds
Fresh blueberries, raspberries or strawberries, to serve
Milk or natural yoghurt, to serve

Method
1. Mix the oats, dried apricots, raisins, dried prunes or dates, Brazil nuts, pumpkin seeds and sunflower seeds together in a bowl.

2. Top with a handful of the berries and pour over the milk or natural yoghurt.

Crunchy green bean, Brazil nut and sesame seed salad (serves one)

In this recipe, the Brazil nuts provide selenium, calcium, magnesium and vitamin B1, while the sesame seeds provide calcium and vitamin B3. The green beans are also a decent source of B vitamins, calcium and magnesium.

Ingredients

75 g trimmed green beans

1 red pepper, deseeded and sliced

2 tbsp fresh coriander, chopped

2 tsp sesame seeds, toasted

30 g Brazil nuts, chopped

4 tbsp extra virgin olive oil

2 tbsp balsamic vinegar

1 tbsp red wine vinegar

1 tsp Dijon mustard

Sea salt and freshly ground black pepper, to taste

Method

1. Place the green beans in a little water and cook in the microwave or simmer gently on the hob until tender. Transfer to a bowl.

2. Stir in the rest of the salad ingredients and season to taste with the sea salt and freshly ground black pepper. Serve with brown crusty bread.

Turkey club sandwich (serves four)

This sandwich contains turkey, granary bread and natural yogurt to keep the blood sugar levels steady and to boost serotonin and B vitamin levels. The natural yogurt also provides calming calcium.

Ingredients

2 tbsp extra virgin olive oil

4 turkey breast steaks

3 tbsp fresh red or green pesto

200 g carton of natural set bio yogurt

1 granary baguette, cut into quarters
4 ripe plum tomatoes, sliced
Small bag of baby leaf salad
Black pepper and sea salt

Method

1. Heat one tablespoon of the extra virgin olive oil in a griddle pan. Season the turkey and cook over a medium heat for 8–10 minutes, turning until browned and cooked right through. Put to one side.

2. Stir the pesto into the natural set bio yogurt and season to taste. Slice each baguette quarter in half lengthways, to make eight halves. Brush the cut sides with the rest of the olive oil, then cook them in the griddle or toast them under a hot grill until they are golden.

3. To make up the sandwiches, spread a little pesto and natural yogurt sauce on four baguette halves, then top with the sliced plum tomatoes. Place the turkey breast on top, then add a handful of salad leaves and another spoonful of the pesto and natural yogurt sauce. Put the other baguette halves on top and serve immediately.

Salmon and rocket pasta (serves four)

This recipe contains salmon, which is rich in omega-3 oil, and rocket, a good source of folate, for healthy brain function. Both the salmon and the wholewheat pasta boost vitamin B complex and serotonin levels and balance the blood sugar. Basil is thought to ease anxiety and chilli helps you relax.

Ingredients

4 skinless and boneless salmon steaks

320 g wholewheat pasta (e.g. spaghetti or penne)

2 garlic cloves

1 red chilli

6 tbsp extra virgin olive oil

80 g rocket

Handful fresh basil leaves, torn

Method

1. Cook the pasta according to the instructions on the packet.

2. Skin and crush the garlic. Peel and finely chop the chilli.

3. Cut the salmon into 2.5-cm cubes.

4. Heat four tablespoons of the extra virgin olive oil in a large frying pan or wok. Add the salmon cubes and cook gently for 3–4 minutes. Add the garlic and chilli to the pan and fry gently until the salmon is cooked.

5. Add the salmon mixture, including the oil it is cooked in, to the drained pasta. Add the rocket, basil and remaining extra virgin olive oil. Toss the ingredients together over a low heat, ensuring that the pasta is hot and well coated in the oil. Serve immediately.

Vegetable chilli (serves four)

This recipe contains brown rice, lentils, kidney beans, mushrooms and natural yoghurt, which help stabilise the blood sugar, boost B vitamin, calcium and magnesium levels and supply tryptophan, which increases serotonin levels. The mushrooms also contain selenium, while the fresh chillies promote relaxation.

Ingredients

320 g brown basmati rice
175 g dried green lentils or one 400 g can lentils
2 tbsp extra virgin olive oil
1 large onion, chopped
1–2 cloves garlic, crushed
1–2 finely chopped red chillies (according to taste)
1 tsp cumin seeds
1 red and 1 green pepper, stalk and seeds removed and chopped
2 carrots, peeled and chopped
2 x 400 g cans chopped tomatoes
1 heaped tbsp tomato purée
300 ml of vegetable stock (make with a stock cube or bouillon powder)
100 g frozen peas
175 g mushrooms, wiped and quartered
1 courgette, chopped
Sea salt and freshly ground black pepper
1 x 400 g can of kidney beans, drained
4 tbsp natural yoghurt
4 tbsp fresh coriander

Method

1. If you are using dried lentils, soak them in boiling water for 30 minutes, then drain. Alternatively, open the canned lentils and drain.

2. Heat the extra virgin olive oil in a large saucepan and fry the onion, garlic, chillies and cumin seeds together, until the onions are soft. Add the peppers, carrots and drained green lentils and cook for 5 minutes, stirring continuously. Add the tomatoes, tomato purée, stock and peas, bring to the boil

and simmer until the lentils are tender. This takes around 30 minutes.

3. In the meantime, cook the brown basmati rice according to the instructions on the packet.

4. Add the mushrooms and courgette to the chilli sauce and simmer for a further 5 minutes. Add seasoning to taste.

5. Finally, add the kidney beans and simmer for another 5 minutes. Spoon the chilli sauce over the cooked and drained brown basmati rice. Top each serving with a tablespoonful of natural yoghurt and fresh coriander.

Jargon Buster

Listed below are the meanings of terms that may be used in connection with anxiety disorders and depression.

Adaptogen – a substance that helps the body adapt to and deal with stress.

Amino acids – organic acids that form the building blocks of proteins.

Cognitive behavioural therapy (CBT) – a treatment that targets negative thought and behaviour patterns.

Dopamine – a neurotransmitter that is involved in feelings of pleasure.

Double-blind – a trial where information that may influence the behaviour of the investigators or the participants is withheld, e.g. which participants have been given a placebo rather than an active substance.

Gamma-aminobutyric acid (GABA) – a neurotransmitter that promotes calm by reducing brain activity.

Glycaemic index (GI) – a ranking of foods according to the effect they have on blood sugar levels.

Hormones – chemicals produced by glands to carry messages to various organs in the body.

Metabolism – physical and chemical processes by which substances are broken down into energy or produced for use in the body.

Neurotransmitter – a brain chemical with a role in the transmission of messages from one nerve cell to another. Some neurotransmitters increase brain activity and others reduce it.

Placebo – an inactive substance given to study participants to compare its effects with those of a treatment, or so that they can benefit from believing they have received a treatment and will therefore feel better.

Precursor – a substance used by the body to produce another substance.

Selenium – a trace mineral that is essential to the body.

Serotonin – a neurotransmitter involved in various bodily functions, including mood, appetite, sleep and sensory perception.

Symmetry – the placing of objects of a similar size and shape at equal distances on opposite sides of an imaginary dividing line.

Tryptophan – an amino acid that is used by the body to make the mood-enhancing neurotransmitter serotonin.

Useful Products

Below is a list of products and suppliers of products that may help ease anxiety. The author doesn't endorse or recommend any particular product and this list is by no means exhaustive.

5-HTP 100 mg
Supplement containing 5-HTP, vitamin C, biotin, niacin, vitamin B6, folic acid and zinc.
  Website: www.healthspan.co.uk

Dendron Stressless
Tablets harnessing the sedative properties of hops, skullcap, valerian and vervain to help relieve stress.
  Website: www.hollandandbarrett.com

Dormeasan
Registered herbal tincture, containing valerian and hops, that relieves stress, calms and relaxes. Provides relief from sleep disturbances caused by the symptoms of mild anxiety.
  Website: www.avogel.co.uk

ESI Passiflora and Valerian Plus
Alcohol-free liquid extract to aid relaxation and sleep. Contains passiflora (passion flower), valerian, Californian poppy, hawthorn and linden.
  Website: www.natural-alternative-products.co.uk

Eurovital GABA Plus

Capsules containing 200 mg of GABA, inositol (vitamin B8) and niacin (vitamin B3) to reduce stress and anxiety, encourage relaxation and promote sleep by reducing nerve cell activity.

Website: www.biovea.com/uk

G Baldwin & Co

Herbalist founded in London in 1844. Offers a wide range of herbal supplements, tinctures and teabags.

Website: www.baldwins.co.uk

Herbs for Healing

A Gloucester-based company with an online shop selling medicinal plants and dried herbs, as well as herbal bath and skin products and the equipment and ingredients to make your own. The website also offers useful information about the medicinal properties of herbs and herbal recipes.

Website: www.herbsforhealing.org.uk

Kalms

A herbal remedy for anxiety, irritability and stress, containing valerian, gentian and hops.

Website: www.kalmsstress.com

Kira LowMood Relief

A herbal supplement containing standardised 450 mg extract of St John's wort.

Website: www.naturalhealthylife.co.uk

Lumie Bodyclock

A clock that helps regulate the sleep–wake cycle by simulating sunrise to waken you gently and naturally.

Website: www.lumie.com

Magnesium B

A supplement containing magnesium, vitamin B complex and vitamin C for a healthy nervous system.

Website: www.wassen.com

Nature's Way Skullcap Herb

Capsules containing skullcap herb. One serving (2 capsules) contains 850 mg of skullcap.

Website: www.natureswayuk.com

Nelsons Homeopathic Pharmacy

Online shop selling homeopathic remedies, including a combination for nervous anxiety that includes arsen alb, aconite and gelsemium. Also sells Bach flower remedies.

Website: www.nelsonshomeopathy.com

Pulse Original Omega-3 Pure Fish Oils with Vitamin E

Capsules containing 260 mg of omega-3 essential fatty acids and vitamin E.

Website: www.seven-seas.com

Relax

A tea containing a blend of organic camomile, fennel and marshmallow root to help calm the nerves and promote relaxation.

Website: www.pukkaherbs.com

RelaxHerb

Supplement containing pharmaceutical grade extract of passion flower to relieve mild anxiety.

Website: www.schwabepharma.co.uk

Salus House Organic Lemon Balm Teabags
Teabags containing lemon balm to soothe the nerves and boost mood.

Website: www.baldwins.co.uk

SAMe tablets by Biovea
Enteric-coated tablets containing 200 mg of SAMe, vitamins B6 and B12, and folic acid.

Website: www.biovea.com/uk

Serotone – 5-HTP
Supplement containing 5-HTP (50 mg/100 mg) along with zinc and B vitamins.

Website: www.highernature.co.uk

Seven Seas Original Pure Cod Liver Oil Liquid
Pure cod liver oil with vitamins A, D and E.

Website: www.seven-seas.com

Skullcap, Oat and Passionflower Compound
A classic nerve tonic containing a range of calming herbs including skullcap, oats, passion flower and valerian.

Website: www.napiers.net

Solgar B-Complex with Vitamin C Stress Formula
Supplement containing ten B vitamins and vitamin C. Free from gluten, wheat and dairy and suitable for vegans.

Website: www.solgar.co.uk

Solgar 5-Hydroxytryptophan (5-HTP)

Supplement containing 100 mg of 5-HTP, along with magnesium, valerian root extract and vitamin B6.

Website: www.solgar.co.uk

Tisserand Aromatherapy

This company offers a wide range of good-quality essential oils.

Website: www.tisserand.com

Vitano Rhodiola Tablets

A supplement containing pharmaceutical grade standardised extract of rhodiola rosea root to relieve mild anxiety, stress and exhaustion.

Website: www.schwabepharma.co.uk

Helpful Books

Amen, Daniel G., *Change Your Brain, Change Your Life: The breakthrough programme for conquering anger, anxiety and depression* (Piatkus, 2009) – this book puts forward a strong argument that many psychological problems, including anxiety disorders, have a biological cause. The author explains how abnormal brain function can be corrected through good nutrition, specific psychological exercises and medication.

Austin, Denise, *Pilates for Every Body: Strengthen, lengthen and tone your body* (Rodale, 2003) – a useful guide to Pilates with various routines lasting 5 or 10 minutes, including ones for beginners.

Bailey, Sue, and Shooter, Mike, *The Young Mind: An essential guide to mental health for young adults, parents and teachers* (Bantam Press, 2009) – helpful information and guidance on mental health issues, including anxiety, that affect children and young people.

Branch, Rhena, and Willson, Rob, *Cognitive Behavioural Therapy for Dummies,* (John Wiley & Sons, second edition, 2010) – a great introduction to CBT and how to use it to help you beat psychological problems, such as anxiety disorders and depression.

Carlson, Richard, *Don't Sweat the Small Stuff… and It's All Small Stuff: Simple ways to keep the little things from taking over your life* (Hodder, 2008) – this book offers some effective strategies to help you achieve inner calm.

Carlson, Richard, *Stop Thinking, Start Living: Discover lifelong happiness* (Element, 2012) – this book explains how happiness is a state of mind and is not dependent on circumstances.

Davis, Patricia, *Aromatherapy: An A–Z: The most comprehensive guide to aromatherapy ever published* (Vermillion, 2005) – a comprehensive guide to essential oils and how to use them to reduce stress and improve your well-being.

Gillanders, Ann, *A Gaia Busy Person's Guide to Reflexology: Simple routines for home, work and travel* (Gaia Books Ltd, 2006) – an indispensable self-help guide to reflexology.

Holford, Patrick, *Optimum Nutrition for the Mind* (Piatkus, 2007) – a useful guide to the foods and supplements that can help relieve mental health issues, including anxiety.

James, Oliver, *Affluenza* (Vermilion, 2007) – this book offers an interesting perspective on the increase in mental health problems, including anxiety, in the UK, contending that excessive materialism is to blame. James suggests that the antidote is to be grateful for what you have and buying what you need rather than what you want.

Margo, Sammy, *The Good Sleep Guide* (Vermilion, 2008) – this book is written by a physiotherapist and includes some good advice on how to select the right pillow and mattress for you to help ensure a comfortable night's sleep.

Weekes, Claire, *Self-help for Your Nerves: Learn to relax and enjoy life again by overcoming stress and fear* (Thorsons, 1995) – a useful guide to overcoming fear and anxiety and becoming more confident.

Directory

The following list of contacts offers information, support and products for sufferers of anxiety disorders.

Action for Happiness

Part of the Young Foundation charity that aims to help people take practical action to improve their mental well-being and to create a happier and more caring society. The website offers a range of self-help resources to help you boost your levels of happiness. The charity's patron is the Dalai Lama.

Website: www.actionforhappiness.org

Anxiety Care UK

A charity based in east London that specialises in helping people recover from anxiety disorders with mutual support groups and structured recovery sessions. The website offers a wide range of information on anxiety, phobias and OCD.

Emotional support: recoveryinfo@anxietycare.org.uk

Website: www.anxietycare.org.uk

Anxiety UK (formerly The National Phobics Society)

A national charity set up in 1970 by an agoraphobic. The website offers information on dealing with anxiety and phobias, as well as a directory of independent self-help groups across the UK. There is also a Stress Tips app with useful tips and advice on managing anxiety. Members can access infoline, email, text and live chat services, as well as therapy and counselling from qualified practitioners face-to-face, over the telephone, or via webcam at reduced rates. Annual membership currently costs £30.

Helpline: 08444 775 774

Email: support@anxietyuk.org.uk

Website: www.anxietyuk.org.uk

Big White Wall

A safe online community of people, guided by trained professionals, who support and help each other by sharing what's troubling them. It is available free in many areas of the UK via the NHS (you can check by typing in your postcode on the website), some employers and universities. It is also free to all UK serving personnel, veterans and their families.

Website: www.bigwhitewall.com

The Body Control Pilates Association

A website offering information about Pilates, a directory of qualified instructors and an online shop.

Email: info@bodycontrol.co.uk

Website: www.bodycontrolpilates.com

The Body Dysmorphic Disorder Foundation

A UK charity that aims to raise awareness and understanding of body dysmorphic disorder. The website offers useful information and resources – including an interactive online questionnaire to help you determine whether you have BDD. There is a directory of BDD support groups – though there are very few. There are also details of online Skype support groups (audio only).

Website: bddfoundation.org

Choose Your Medication

A website offering up-to-date information by UK experts about mental health conditions, UK licensed drug treatments and their side effects. Its aim is to help people make informed decisions about medications used in the mental health setting.

Website: www.chooseyourmedication.org

Citizens Advice Bureau

Helps people resolve their legal, financial, emotional and other problems by providing free, independent and confidential advice. Visit the website for online advice, webchat and contact details for your local branch.

Website: www.citizensadvice.org.uk

Cruse Bereavement Care

Promotes the well-being of bereaved people and helps them understand their grief and cope with their loss. Provides support and offers information, advice, education and training services.

Helpline: 0844 477 9400
Email: helpline@cruse.org.uk
Website: www.cruse.org.uk

Depression Alliance

A charity offering support to sufferers of depression through publications, videos and self-help groups. Also campaigns to end the stigma of depression and to raise awareness of what it means to live with it.

Website: www.depressionalliance.org

Depression UK

A charity that promotes mutual support between people with or at risk from depression, to encourage self-help, recovery and personal growth. Members' services include penfriend and phone-friend schemes, an information phoneline and an online discussion forum. The current annual membership fee is £10.

Email: info@depressionuk.org

Website: www.depressionuk.org

Do You Panic

A website created by Will Beswick, who uses his own experience of recovering from anxiety to help other sufferers.

Website: www.doyoupanic.co.uk

e-couch

A free online programme that provides information about emotional problems, including what causes them, how to prevent them and how to treat them. It includes exercises and strategies to help you understand yourself and others better.

Website: ecouch.anu.edu.au

Emetophobia Help

A website, set up by a sufferer of emetophobia (fear of vomiting), who is also a registered counsellor, to provide information for others with the condition, including a fact sheet and a blog. You can email for a refundable mentoring session via Skype.

Email: annachristie@shaw.ca

Website: www.emetophobiahelp.org

Flying without Fear

Flying without fear is a one-day course run by Virgin Atlantic to help people overcome their fear of flying.

Website: www.flyingwithoutfear.co.uk

Food and Mood

Explores the relationship between what you eat and how you feel, and offers tips on how to incorporate healthy eating into your life.

Website: www.mind.org.uk/foodandmood

Food for the Brain

A charity that aims to promote the link between optimum nutrition and mental health. It offers nutritional advice, a free monthly e-newsletter, an online cognitive function test and up-to-date information on diet and mental health.

Website: www.foodforthebrain.org

Food Intolerance Awareness

A division of Allergy UK set up to help people identify whether they have a food intolerance. It provides useful information, including a food and symptoms diary to help you determine whether you suffer from food intolerance and which foods are your triggers.

Website: www.foodintoleranceawareness.org

The Happiness Project

This was founded by psychologist Dr Robert Holden and aims to help people find happiness by changing the way they think. It also offers courses in happiness and positivity. The website includes inspiring quotes and articles, and an online happiness test.

Website: www.robertholden.org

Health Supplements Information Service

Service that aims to provide accurate and balanced information on vitamins, minerals and food supplements.

Website: www.hsis.org

The International Stress Management Association

A registered charity with a multi-disciplinary professional membership that includes the UK and the Republic of Ireland. It exists to promote sound knowledge and best practice in the prevention and reduction of human stress and provides referrals to stress management professionals. The website offers free factsheets and a stress questionnaire.

Website: www.isma.org.uk

Living Life to the Full

A website offering a free online life skills course (based on CBT) that is supported by the NHS and is especially helpful to people suffering from anxiety or depression. The course is written by Dr Chris Williams, a senior lecturer in psychiatry, and includes training in controlling anxiety.

Website: www.llttf.com

Medicines and Healthcare products Regulatory Agency (MHRA)

A government agency responsible for ensuring that medicines and medical devices work and are acceptably safe. The website includes a section on the safety of herbal medicines and a full list of herbal medicines that have been granted a traditional herbal registration (THR).

Website: www.mhra.gov.uk

Mental Health Foundation

A UK charity that provides helpful information and carries out research on the causes, prevention and treatment of mental health problems, including anxiety and anxiety-related disorders. The foundation also campaigns for and works to improve services for anyone affected by mental health problems. It takes an integrated approach to mental health that incorporates both social and biological factors. Online resources include downloadable podcasts on various topics, including how to overcome fear and anxiety, and stress management techniques. The charity's Be Mindful campaign offers information on mindfulness, including a mindfulness exercise and details of mindfulness courses in the UK.

Websites: www.mentalhealth.org.uk; bemindful.co.uk

Mental Health Matters

A national charity that provides a variety of services to help people with mental health needs.

Website: www.mentalhealthmatters.com

Mind

A national charity for people with emotional and mental health problems, including anxiety. Offers information and advice online and through a network of local Mind associations. The charity also provides two confidential mental health information services, the Mind Infoline and the Legal Advice Service.

Mind Infoline: 0300 123 3393 – 9 a.m.–6 p.m., Monday–Friday, (except for bank holidays)

Text Infoline: 86463

Email: info@mind.org.uk

Website: www.mind.org.uk

MoodGYM

A website, developed by the National Institute of Mental Health Research at the Australian National University, that offers a free CBT-based training programme to help users deal with mental health issues, including GAD and depression.

   Website: www.moodgym.anu.edu.au

Moodjuice

A website developed by Choose Life Falkirk and the Adult Clinical Psychology Service, NHS Forth Valley. It offers information and advice to those experiencing troublesome thoughts, feelings and actions. The site offers self-help guides on various psychological issues, including anxiety, stress, panic, depression and sleep problems. You can also explore various aspects of your life that may be causing you distress.

   Website: www.moodjuice.scot.nhs.uk

The National Association for Premenstrual Syndrome

A charity offering information and advice to women who suffer from PMS. Services offered include expert advice, a monthly e-bulletin, an online forum and an online menstrual diary to help you and your GP determine whether you have PMS.

   Website: www.pms.org.uk

National Debtline

Offers free confidential and independent advice on how to deal with debt problems. The website offers useful resources to help you deal with debt, including a four-step self-help guide, an interactive debt advice tool and an online budget form.

   Freephone: 0808 808 4000 – Monday–Friday, 9 a.m.–9 p.m. and Saturday, 9.30 a.m.–1 p.m.

   Website: www.nationaldebtline.co.uk

NHS Choices

An NHS website that aims to help you make choices about your health, from decisions about your lifestyle, such as smoking, drinking and exercise, to finding and using NHS services in England. There is a section called Moodzone which aims to help people cope with stress, anxiety and depression by providing useful information, interactive tools, and videos and real-life stories. You can also find out about psychological therapy services, such as counselling and CBT, near you.

Useful online tools include workplace stress, depression and food allergies self-assessments and 'mental health' and 'lift your mood' video walls, where people share their experiences via video clips. There are also blogs and forums on specific health topics (NHS Choices Talk), including mental health issues, such as anxiety disorders and depression.

Website: www.nhs.uk

No Panic

A voluntary charity that offers information, advice and support. as well as various booklets, CDs, DVDs and books, to help sufferers deal with their condition.

Helpline: 0844 967 4848 (every day, 10 a.m.–10 p.m.; service charge: 5 p a minute)

Youth helpline: 01753 840393 (for 13–20 year olds, open 4 p.m.–6 p.m, Monday–Friday)

Website: www.nopanic.org.uk

OCD Action

A national charity for people with OCD and related disorders. The charity provides information, advice and support for sufferers and their family, friends and carers, and promotes awareness and understanding of OCD and related disorders. Online resources include a self-assessment for OCD.

Help and information line: 0845 390 6232

Email: support@ocdaction.org.uk

Website: www.ocdaction.org.uk

OCD-UK

A charity set up in 2003 by two OCD sufferers who felt that the condition was not widely recognised. The organisation provides information, as well as practical and emotional support, for OCD sufferers, including an advice line, community support forums and support groups.

Advice line: 0845 120 3778

Email: support@ocduk.org

Website: www.ocduk.org

OCD Youth

A website set up by the Maudsley Hospital Clinic for Young People with OCD that provides useful information and advice for young people with OCD.

Website: ocdyouth.iop.kcl.ac.uk/youngpeople/

Patient UK Experience

Online forums run by Patient UK, a website that offers 'comprehensive health information as provided by GPs and nurses to patients during consultations'. Forum topics include anxiety disorders.

Website: experience.patient.co.uk

The Phobia List

A website providing a comprehensive A–Z of phobias.

Website: www.phobialist.com

Relate

With 2,500 professionally trained counsellors, Relate is the UK's largest provider of relationship counselling and sex therapy. Offers counselling, sex therapy and relationship education to support couple and family relationships throughout life. Visit the website to find your nearest Relate or to consult a counsellor by email or talk to a counsellor live online via live chat. Alternatively, you can arrange counselling by telephone.

Website: www.relate.org.uk

Relaxation for Living Institute

Offers courses, DVDs and CDs that aim to teach people how to relax and deal with stress and anxiety using breathing and muscle relaxation techniques.

Website: www.rfli.co.uk

Rethink

A mental health charity offering information on mental health issues, including anxiety disorders, and a variety of support services, including support groups, and advice and helplines.

Advice and information service: 0300 5000 927 (10 a.m.–2 p.m., Monday–Friday)

Website: www.rethink.org

The Royal College of Psychiatrists

The Royal College of Psychiatrists is the professional and educational body for psychiatrists in the United Kingdom and the Republic of Ireland. It aims to set standards and promote excellence in psychiatry and mental healthcare. The website offers information on a wide range of mental health issues, including anxiety, panic, phobias, OCD, stress and depression.

Website: www.rcpsych.ac.uk

Samaritans

Offers confidential non-judgemental emotional support, 24 hours a day, to people experiencing feelings of distress or despair, including those that could lead to suicide. This service is available over the telephone, by email, by letter or face to face; you can find details of your nearest local branch on the website. At the time of writing this book, the charity also plans to introduce text support and online support services in the near future.

Address: Freepost RSRB-KKBY-CYJK, PO Box 9090, Stirling, FK8 2SA

Telephone: 116 123

Email: jo@samaritans.org

Website: www.samaritans.org

Sane

A charity that offers information and support to people affected by mental illness and conducts research into mental illness. There is an online support forum and a textcare support service as well as a telephone helpline.

Helpline: 0300 304 7000 (daily, 6 p.m.–11 p.m.)

Email: sanemail@org.uk

Website: www.sane.org.uk

See Me

See Me is Scotland's Programme to tackle mental health stigma and discrimination. The charity is funded by Scottish Government and Comic Relief and is managed by the Scottish Association for Mental Health (SAMH) and the Mental Health Foundation. It campaigns to end the discrimination and stigma attached to mental ill-health.

Website: www.seemescotland.org

Smokefree

An NHS website offering advice and support to help quit smoking. You can choose from a range of support options, including your local stop smoking service, as well as email, text and online chat support services.

Smokefree national helpline: 0300 123 1044

Website: www.nhs.uk/smokefree

Social Anxiety UK

Founded in March 2000 by a group of social anxiety sufferers after learning that there were no UK-based websites for people with social anxiety problems. The organisation offers information and advice for sufferers and a range of support services, including an online forum and chatrooms.

Website: www.social-anxiety.org.uk

The Stress Management Society

The Stress Management Society is a non-profit-making organisation dedicated to helping people tackle stress. Website offers information on stress-management techniques such as self-hypnosis and self-massage. The society also offers a free e-newsletter, an online stress coaching tool and stress-management workshops.

Website: www.stress.org.uk

Talkmentalhealth

An online discussion forum run by Talkhealth Partnership, a leading UK social health community, providing online information on a range of conditions.

Website: www.talkhealth.com/talkmentalhealth

Triumph Over Phobia

Triumph Over Phobia (TOP UK) is a UK-registered charity that aims to help sufferers of phobias, obsessive compulsive disorder and other anxiety-related conditions to overcome their fears through a network of self-help therapy groups.

Website: www.topuk.org

Women's Health Concern

A charity offering online information on women's health issues, including PMS and the menopause. Also offers email and telephone advice, and holds conferences and seminars.

Website: www.womens-health-concern.org

YoungMinds

A UK charity committed to improving the emotional well-being and mental health of children and young people. Raises awareness of children and young people's mental health and provides expert knowledge through training, outreach work, publications and a telephone helpline for parents and carers.

Parents' helpline: 0808 802 5544 (Monday–Friday, 9.30 a.m.–4 p.m (freephone))

Website: www.youngminds.org.uk

IBS

A self-help guide to feeling better

Wendy Green

Foreword by Dr Nick Read,
chair of The IBS Network

IBS
A self-help guide to feeling better

Wendy Green

£8.99
Paperback
ISBN: 978-1-84953-807-7

In this easy-to-follow book, Wendy Green explains how food intolerances, gut infections and bacterial imbalance, and stress and hormones contribute to IBS, and offers practical advice and a holistic approach to help you deal with the symptoms, including simple dietary and lifestyle changes, and DIY complementary therapies. Find out 50 things you can do today to help you cope with IBS, including:

- ▶ Identify your IBS triggers and learn how to manage them
- ▶ Choose beneficial foods and supplements
- ▶ Manage stress and relax to reduce flare-ups
- ▶ Discover practical tips for living with IBS
- ▶ Adopt preventative strategies
- ▶ Find helpful organisations and products

Have you enjoyed this book?
If so, why not write a review on your favourite website?

If you're interested in finding out more about our books, find
us on Facebook at **Summersdale Publishers** and follow us on
Twitter at **@Summersdale**.

Thanks very much for buying this Summersdale book.

www.summersdale.com